From

OVERWHELMED

to

Inspired

From

OVERWHELMED

to

Inspired

YOUR PERSONAL GUIDE TO HEALTH AND WELL-BEING

Mary Jayne Rogers Ph.D.

ISBN-13: **9781534853089**
ISBN-10: **1534853081**
Library of Congress Control Number: **2016910481**
CreateSpace Independent Publishing Platform
North Charleston, South Carolina

Dedication

This book is dedicated to you and to the power you have to change the world, one small step at a time.

Contents

Forward by Cedric Bryant

In our busy, time-constrained culture where multi-tasking reigns supreme, it is rare that we take the time to focus on ourselves. So, when a book is published complete with simple, meaningful approaches for helping us improve the quality of our lives, it's worthwhile to read it. In *From Overwhelmed to Inspired*, Mary Jane Rogers, encourages the reader to begin a journey toward a lifetime of wellness through practicing what she calls the "Three Essentials to Wellness," (1) the "3 Selfs" (i.e., self-esteem, self-respect, self-efficacy), (2) compassion for the self and others, and (3) mindful awareness. Dr. Rogers points out that throughout this journey, we must always be mindful of our individuality and how we can best attend to our specific needs. The book also gives Dr. Roger's take on making the best choices for health with an easy-to-remember acronym, OWN: Oxygen, Water, and Nourishment. These choice-related topic areas deal with breathing and movement, hydration, and nutrition. For the reader interested in developing wellness, Dr. Rogers states, "It is a worthwhile journey. Let's take it together, one step at a time."

Dr. Rogers delivers on her intention to help others successfully progress toward wellness by offering tools to help you understand what wellness means to you, information to make better choices for yourself and your family, and strategies that are easy to incorporate, simple to understand, and fun. This eloquently written book details the author's powerful personal story about her struggles as an adolescent and adult dealing with body-images issues and how those experiences have guided her focus on her path to wellness. This book has all of the components to help those of us who could use practical advice on improving our lives through improved wellness, and reminds us that it is definitely worth the effort.

Cedric X. Bryant, Ph.D., FACSM
Chief Science Officer
American Council on Exercise

Preface

THE JOURNEY BEGINS

"Are you in earnest? Then seize
*   this very minute.*
What you can do, or dream you can, begin it.
Boldness has genius and magic in it;
*   only engage then the mind grows heated;*
Begin, and then the work will be completed."

~ *GOETHE*

Dear Traveling Companion,
As with any journey, we all begin somewhere.

I have struggled for years with food and disordered eating and exercise.

I was a quiet, introverted little girl in a family that suffered tumultuous times with alcoholism and divorce. Movement and play gave me solace and allowed me to discover a piece of myself that I could own. They brought me freedom, joy and exhilaration. I recognized very early on that imaginative movement was my refuge, a magic carpet that transported me to a place that was all mine; where I was a winner; talented and important. It was fantastic - until that life altering day down the road when, like a Mac truck, it hit me – *puberty*. With it, like most teenaged girls, adolescence brought fear that I didn't fit in; that my changing body didn't conform to the ideal image that society, as described by the magazine covers of the day, deemed as beautiful – or even acceptable. Right in the middle of all of this normal teenage turmoil, fate waved her wry wand when I was required to participate in a swimsuit contest as part of a regional Key Club event, (yes, like a traditional beauty pageant). You can imagine the introverted little girl and the fears that came to the surface at the thought of being exposed and potentially publicly rejected. It was right about that time that I became acutely aware that my super-skinny boyfriend wore blue jeans that were smaller than mine. Through my distorted lens I began to see my adolescent curves as unwelcome fat. To this day, I wincingly recoil from the memory of parading around in a bikini, being judged by a pack of hormonal teenage boys.

I convinced myself that if I weighed 90 pounds, I would have the perfect body and not only fit into my boyfriend's jeans, but have them be a bit baggy. Hello, disordered eating and exercise behavior! Movement was no longer my refuge. It was my jailer. I obsessed about calorie consumption and exercise. I refused to eat more than 250 calories a day and spent every free moment exercising. As time went on, I eventually discovered that if I "purged" with laxatives or vomiting, I could have occasional meals or family celebrations and still remain loyal to my distorted lifestyle.

Through the years I tried practically every kind of diet, from Atkins, to cabbage soup, to grapefruit, to brown rice. When I was not on a "diet", I was eating ridiculously low calories or eating too much and purging. These behaviors lasted into my 20's, well into graduate school and marriage. Back in those days, the concept of eating disorders was a barely known phenomenon. In the beginning, I had no idea that my behavior was dysfunctional. In fact, some of my friends and family who were struggling with weight loss actually applauded my will power.

As the years went on, inconsistent with my private eating and exercise behaviors, I was pursuing an advanced degree in exercise physiology. Intellectually, I knew there was something wrong with me. My mother had a friend who died of unknown causes. For some reason she just quit eating. Over many months and with a great deal of introspection, I recognized that my behaviors were not at all healthy and indeed quite harmful, but I was ashamed to admit my behaviors to others and, of course, I was afraid of gaining weight. Ironically, I was heavier and carrying more fat than ever.

The turning point came when my husband and I decided to start a family. I knew I couldn't continue these behaviors and maintain a healthy pregnancy. And, so it was that I quietly and privately set out with a plan to overcome the noxious way of dealing with food and exercise and begin a new conversation with food, activity and my body.

Since then, it has been my calling to search for answers about how to achieve optimal health and well-being and to share what I have learned with others.

What about you? Where does your journey begin? Each of us comes to this place from our own personal experiences. But along the way we've developed feelings and attitudes about food and exercise, whether we recognize it or not. How we deal with these feelings affects our overall health and well-being.

Through my experience I have learned that unhealthy relationships with food, exercise and body image don't have a "cure" – no matter what people say. Unlike alcoholism or drug addiction, in which sufferers can find sanctuary in abstinence, those of us who struggle in our relationship with food and exercise cannot simply stop eating and moving. Our bodies NEED healthy food and mindful movement not just to survive, but to thrive. That means that every day, every meal, every snack, indeed – every bite- is a choice to move in the direction of a healthy mind, healthy spirit and healthy body.

This is NOT a diet and exercise book. It is the beginning of a journey toward a lifetime of wellness. I hope you will accept it as my heartfelt desire to help you find meaningful solutions to the questions, craziness and overwhelming information about how we find our way to this thing called wellness. As we go along we will discover that making better choices to experience a more healthful life will bring exuberance, happiness and a lifetime of feeling better. When you feel better, you will radiate positive energy to the people around you and they, in turn, will want to feel the glow of health as well. In this way, choice by choice, you begin to change your life and the lives of those around you. In this simple but profound way, you have the power to make a difference in the world. It is a worthwhile journey. Let's take it together, one step at a time.

"The journey of a thousand miles begins with one step."

~ LAO TZU

Introduction

STEP 1 – DESTINATION WELLNESS. WHERE DO WE BEGIN?

"The part can never be well unless the whole is well."

~ PLATO.

To figure out how to get someplace, we have to know where we're going. Even Dorothy knew she was headed toward Oz. The same is true of our journey toward wellness. What exactly is "wellness"? According to the New York Times, the term can be traced back to the 1650's. While the word itself is over 350 years old, it has only been in the last two decades that wellness found its way into our everyday vocabulary. Even though we recognize and use the word regularly, does anyone really agree on what it means? It is generally presumed that wellness is simply the "opposite of sickness". If you take a moment and consider what wellness looks like to you, I think we can agree wellness is much more than that.

This is evidenced by the fact that billions of dollars are spent/made each year in exercise equipment, diets, supplements, various exercise regimens and other "miracles" aimed at making us slim, healthy, fit and "well". Yet, our nation, as a whole, is sicker, fatter, and further from the concept of "well" than we've ever been.

What does it really mean to "be well"? As a society, we have drifted so far from "well" or "wellness" that we don't even know we have become lost. Looking back at my own experience, I was relatively fit and certainly didn't weigh much. I was not suffering from a physical illness. But I was definitely not well! My skin was constantly erupting, my hair was brittle, my eyes were dull, my digestion was a mess and I was exhausted!

Do any of these things sound familiar to you? When we experience wellness, our skin glows, our eyes sparkle, our hair shines and we have plenty of energy to get through the day. Wellness is the place where we discover that we CAN feel better, live better and *thrive*.

To really grasp the concept of wellness, we must first recognize and accept that we are all different. We are each as unique as snowflakes or grains of sand on the beach. Consequently, what may be absolute wellness for you may not fit the bill for me. This is an important idea to remember going forward. As we move forward, you will begin to notice this concept showing up in your everyday life. Perhaps you will have an "Ahah!" moment when you are talking about trends in health and wellness with your friends and family. You may think, "That idea may work for some people, but it is not my idea of wellness."

Below is a definition of wellness that has always resonated with me:

> *"Wellness - It's the best in each of us, a natural mix of elements that makes us unique. Wellness is a conscious commitment to growth and improvement in all areas. Only then does the larger picture emerge."*
>
> *~ ANONYMOUS*

This *larger picture* is what happens when we begin to realize that we are miraculous creatures made up of billions of bits; cells that are ceaselessly working, striving for harmony to enable us to create our own personal masterpiece. As we attend to our personal wellness, we become healthy and clear minded. Then, a marvelous thing happens. We begin to accomplish more as individuals and therefore also as a society. Our contribution to the greater good, our "picture" enlarges.

Another important thing to note about wellness is that it is not a destination. It is a journey. Throughout our lives, we change; our situations change. We grow. We age. We experience life. As we do these things, our wellness needs and our experience of wellness will change. But throughout this journey, we must always be mindful of *our individuality* and how we can best attend to our specific wellness needs.

In this book I will give you the tools you need to understand what wellness means to you, provide you with the information you need to make better choices for yourself and your family, and do it in a way that is easy to incorporate, simple to understand and fun!

Truly, wellness is not as hard or complex as it has been made out to be. There are basically Three Essentials to Wellness. These are your foundation. With them, the rest is purely a matter of informed choices.

THREE ESSENTIALS TO WELLNESS

(Drum roll please)

1. The "3 Selfs" (Self Esteem, Self Respect, Self Efficacy)
2. Compassion (for Self and Others)
3. Mindful Awareness (Being in the moment)

We will be talking about each of these in detail as we get into the next section of the book. For now, you can set your mind at ease and know that the basics of wellness are straightforward and within reach.

HOW TO GET THE MOST OUT OF THIS BOOK

The book is divided into sections: Mind, Body, Spirit and Stepping Stones. This is *your* journey. You are in control and can begin it wherever you wish. You may be so eager to get started that you want to go straight to the Body section, do that first and then come back around to the Mind section or the Spirit section. However, the sections of the book are arranged in sequence. Each section builds on the knowledge and skills you have gained in previous sections. The skills you practice in the Mind section lay the foundation for the rest of the book. I encourage you begin at the beginning, allow the book to take you step by step and enjoy the ride.

Along the road you will find places to stop and practice what you are learning. You may write your practice notes in the book itself or you may prefer to keep a journal or even a simple spiral notebook to record your thoughts and ideas. Some people prefer to get all the way through the book and then go back a second time to do the practices. Others stop and explore the practices as they go. The most important thing is to actually take time to do the practices as best you can. Words are cheap. It is in the doing that we find progress toward lasting change. The practices allow you to "try on" the topics we are discussing to determine where you are in your process and what works for you. If you struggle, please know that is normal. Try to go a little deeper. Take some extra time and examine what is stalling you. I promise it will be worth the effort.

HOW DO YOU KNOW IF YOU ARE READY?

"It's not that some people have willpower and some do not. It's that some people are ready for change and others are not."

~ JAMES GORDON

This is a good place for our first activity: Determining Your "Readiness."

In the psychology of change, there is a concept called READINESS. We will not change behaviors until we are psychologically READY to do so. The general "readiness scale" tells us where we are on a scale ranging from:

(i)   Not ready to change;
(ii)   Weighing the pros and cons;
(iii) Making small changes here and there;
(iv) Already changing;
(v)   Making it a lifestyle.

The good news is you are reading this right now, which indicates that at the very least you are at the stage, weighing the pros and cons. Continuing with the book will help you to move further along the "readiness scale" and to make changes as you go that will lead you to lifetime wellness. The readiness scale takes into account that we all have times in our lives when we aren't as on track as we would like to be in our journey to a healthier lifestyle. These setbacks are known as lapses, and even lapses are built in to the readiness profile. Along the way we will talk about being aware of setbacks and strategies to get back on track. As we travel this road together, I will share with you my journey through the readiness scale. Even after all these years, I still experience lapses. These are the times that the information and practices in the MIND section see me through and will see you through as well. With that in mind, it's time to figure out your starting point. Where you are you on the "readiness scale"?

PRACTICE

To assess where you are on the Readiness Scale, begin here.

Which Stage of Readiness are you in? (circle one)

1. Not Ready (This is not you!)
2. Weighing the Pros & Cons (Are you contemplating a change?)
3. Making Small Changes Here & There (Still undecided but seeking out more information)
4. Already Changing (Practicing small changes for a few months and have a strong desire to make permanent changes)
5. Making it a Lifestyle (Feeling good about the changes you have made over the last 6 months and coping with lapses fairly successfully.

Once you have determined your readiness, take a few moments to think about how you decided where you are on the Readiness Scale. In the space below, jot down how you came to this decision and one or two ideas you feel could help you get to the next Stage of Readiness. *(Hint: one might be reading this book!)* As you go through the book, you can refer back to this page to see where you are and how far you've come. You can do this as often as you like.

Notes:

PRACTICE

Take a look at the following questions and jot down your responses. Your answers can help you identify the direction you will take on your journey. Remember, your answers can evolve as you go along. This is just to help you get started.

What is a life change or goal that inspires you?

What area(s) of your life are you most eager to change or improve?

Now take a few moments to sit with your answers. Do they resonate with you? Do they motivate you? If so, you are ready to begin. Turn the page and let's get started!

"Life isn't about finding yourself. Life is about creating yourself."

~ GEORGE BERNARD SHAW

Section 1

Mind

The mind is everything. What you think you become.

~ BUDDHA

When you hear the word wellness, what comes to mind? Weight loss? Exercise? Following a specific diet and exercise regimen perhaps? Most of us, when we think of wellness, tend to focus on our physical selves and all the "doing" required to achieve this thing we think of as *wellness*. But we are more than what we do. In fact, what we do stems from what we think. What we think, as Buddha reminds us, we become. This is the reason we want to start on our wellness journey by planting the seeds of wellness in our imagination. Begin now to imagine what wellness is for you. How might wellness feel?

Hold on to that thought as we enter into the MIND section. Here we will explore the connection between one's thoughts and the experience of wellness. Understanding this relationship will help you to have a deeper appreciation for your journey to wellness and to perhaps feel more at ease along the way.

Remember our definition of wellness: **"Wellness - It's the best in each of us, a natural mix of elements that makes us unique. Wellness is _a conscious commitment_ to growth and improvement in all areas. Only then does the larger picture emerge."**

~ ANONYMOUS

1

"...Wellness is a <u>conscious commitment</u>..."

Why is the word "conscious" so important to our definition of wellness? We can't really *just start* being well. It requires awareness, thought and processing. We must be willing to examine our beliefs and attitudes. Being conscious forces us to make decisions and to think about the decisions we have made.

Wellness also requires commitment. A commitment is a pledge. It implies something thought out and planned; an obligation or responsibility.

Awareness, thought, processing and planning; these are all mental activities. This is not to suggest that the mind and body are separate. In fact, as we go along, we will look at various components of wellness and discover that one's mind and body are one entity, fundamentally related in how they function and respond to the world. But for the sake of organization, let's discuss them in separate sections.

Our MIND section is divided into the segments of the Three Essentials of Wellness: The "Three Selfs", Compassion and Mindful Awareness.

The "Three Selfs" include:

- Self Esteem, which deals with how we feel about ourselves.
- Self Respect, which has to do with possessing a sense of honor or dignity.
- "Self E" or self efficacy, which is our belief in our ability to accomplish a task.

We will consider compassion to be a profound awareness of the suffering of others along with the desire to relieve it and Mindful Awareness as being deeply perceptive of the activities and emotions in the world around you without making judgments.

Let's take each one separately and discuss why they are fundamental to your personal vision of wellness.

1

Wellness Essential #1: The "*Three Selfs*"

Self Esteem - Self Respect -"Self E"

Trust yourself. Create the kind of self that you will be happy to live with all your life. Make the most of yourself by fanning the tiny, inner sparks of possibility into flames of achievement.

~ GOLDA MEIR

Living well is really all about YOU; being aware of yourself, loving yourself, believing in yourself, respecting yourself - nurturing your Self.

The Three Selfs have to do with how we think about ourselves and interact with our world. They are fundamentally important to our ability to achieve a sense of health and well-being.

While they are interrelated and sound similar to one another, they are each distinct and their distinctions make each one relevant to our journey toward healthier, happier lives. Let's take a look:

Self #1. Self Esteem has to do with ***our feelings*** of self-worth; *how we feel about ourselves*. Self esteem envelops us like our personal weather. Like weather, it can fluctuate dramatically from day to day, even moment to moment, as we constantly evaluate ourselves, including our thoughts, behaviors and actions. We have sunny days when we are feeling pretty darn good about ourselves and cloudy days when we feel we could or should be better. Then there are the downright rainy days that pour over us and we feel completely incapable. You can imagine your self esteem as your private weather vane that can point to "feel good about yourself" or flip around in a storm and point to "guilt, shame or worthlessness".

Early in my career in the fitness industry, I had a goal to win a prestigious award that was bestowed by our industry's international organization. It was highly coveted among my peers and required a huge amount of accomplishment and documented success in multiple arenas. The application process was arduous and the competition fierce. I applied three years in a row. The first year I made finalist, but didn't win. My self esteem meter pointed directly to inferior and rejected; very cloudy that day. The second year I made finalist, but once again I didn't win. I felt unworthy. My self esteem had rain that day! The third year – I won! I should have felt sunny right? Not exactly. My shaky self esteem was like rolling thunder that kept me doubting whether I was deserving of the award or if they just gave it to me to get me to stop applying. It wasn't until I gave my acceptance speech that the weather vane of self esteem began to turn. I was able to speak from my heart about an industry I believed in. I received a standing ovation and I could see that my bosses were proud. At last I felt deserving, accomplished and accepted by my industry and my peers. In that moment the fickle weather vane of self esteem pointed to gloriously sunny!

The point is that self esteem deals with how we feel at any given moment, depending on our feelings about the situation we are facing. Understanding and fostering a foundation of strong self esteem helps us to lessen the moments of clouds and rain; we are better able to withstand the darker moments and emerge once again to feeling sunny about ourselves. When we feel good about ourselves, as we do with positive self esteem, we are more likely to make choices that are healthful and constructive. That's why positive self esteem is foundational to the Three Essentials of Wellness.

PRACTICE:

What about you? Can you think of a time when your self esteem felt exceptionally high? What was the circumstance? What are some words that describe how you felt? Close your eyes and allow your body to remember the sensation that you felt when your self esteem was high? If you can't remember a time (many of us can't) try to imagine what it would feel like.

In the space below, write a few words that describe your feelings of high self esteem:

Self #2. Self Respect has its roots in Self Esteem. But here we are making the distinction between *feeling good about* ourselves and *acting in a manner that we believe is deserving of respect*, which in turn promotes a high level of self regard. It has to do with character, dignity, substance and determination.

When we consider what it means to respect others, we recognize in them certain qualities that cause them to be deserving of respect. In turn, these are the qualities that we will see in ourselves that make us feel deserving of respect.

PRACTICE:

Think of a person or persons for whom you have great respect. They can be a living figure or a person who has already passed. What are some of the qualities that come to mind that cause you to respect them? Here are some ideas to get you started: integrity, strong values, compassion for others, or a great ability to overcome challenges. Are there more descriptors you can think of? Jot them down below:

> *Self Respect is demonstrated by our actions. When we respect ourselves, we behave in ways that demonstrate the qualities we listed above. It is an internal appreciation for actions and behaviors that are worthy of respect. As a result, it can often demand that we make difficult choices.*

Now consider yourself. What level of respect do you have for yourself? Can you think of a time that you embodied those characteristics of being worthy of respect? Perhaps a time when you showed great leadership, demonstrated integrity, or overcame a particularly challenging obstacle?

In the space below, write down at least one time when you acted in a way that demonstrated respect for yourself.

When you think back on these events, how did your actions make you feel? Here are some words to help you get started: proud, honorable, strong, trustworthy, honest. What others can you think of?

When you think of these words and events, can you remember the feeling inside your body and your mind that they created? Close your eyes and take a moment and try to recreate that feeling now.

TREATING OURSELVES WITH RESPECT

When we respect others, we dignify them with our words and actions. We certainly are considerate of their feelings. We would never berate them, call them names, or refuse to help if they needed something. That would be "disrespectful". And yet, we do that to ourselves all too frequently.

We may say to ourselves, for example, that we are fat, stupid or lazy. Outwardly this lack of self respect manifests when we use other veiled, self-deprecating phrases; saying things like:

"I was never smart enough to do ___ (Fill in the Blank)___,
"I have never been physically attractive. Boys (Girls) don't like me.
"I don't care about winning. I am just not competitive in that way."
"It doesn't matter what I eat. I have always been like this."
"My brother was the athletic one."
"I just can't do math."
"My sister was the cute, petite one."
"I have always been slow."
"My sister was the smart one in the family."
Are there others you can think of? Jot them down below.

Here is one I caught myself saying to myself the other day, "I don't like these pants. They make my butt look big." Ok, that was bad enough, but then my brain added, *"..well that wouldn't be too difficult."*

Generally, these thoughts or comments emerge unconsciously, but they are disrespectful and unhelpful to our aspiration of feeling better. A more respectful way for me to speak to myself would be to simply acknowledge, "I don't like the way these pants fit."

We are often taught that using self deprecating words and phrases like these are a positive characteristic and demonstrate humility. But in fact, we may say these things about ourselves publicly to discourage others from directing mean comments our way; beat them to the punch so to speak. We really have to remind ourselves that humility is simply modesty, not self-deprecation, and can be expressed in respectful ways.

When we use these words silently to ourselves, we are harming ourselves in two ways. First, we are clawing away at whatever self respect we do possess. Second, we are being unkind and even downright mean. This is not the way someone worthy of respect behaves. So not only are we tearing down what self esteem we already have, we are acting in a way that is not deserving of respect, thus assuring our self respect remains stunted.

PRACTICE:

During conversations with friends, family and coworkers, try to listen for words and phrases that do not support self respect. Once you begin to iden-tify these tendencies in others, perhaps you will begin to notice when you speak unkindly about yourself. When you catch yourself in this pattern, ask yourself why. Why are you using words and phrases that are disrespectful to the most important person in your life – you? There may be many answers to this question. It may make you feel uneasy to examine this. But once you recognize these tendencies and identify their roots, you can choose to avoid language that is disrespectful. Often the most respectful thing you can do is to show kindness to yourself and recognize there can be beauty and respect in silence.

Self #3. "Self E". We have talked about the concept of self esteem dealing with how *we feel* about ourselves and self respect dealing with how we *demonstrate* our worth by our *actions*. Our *"Self E"* concept stands for *Self Efficacy*. "Self E" deals with *our belief in our ability* to accomplish a task or a goal. We are taught about "Self E" as small children. The grown-ups in our lives have encouraged us by saying, "Come on – you can do it!" Or we may have heard the reverse, something like "That's too hard for you," or "You are not strong enough to do that". Some of us have even heard things like, "You will never amount to anything" or "It's better to give up now. Don't waste your time."

Unfortunately, messages such as these from parents, siblings or teachers can stick with us for a lifetime. The types of messages we received as children will impact how we feel about our ability to accomplish any variety of goals, ranging from finishing our education to learning to play a musical instrument.

PRACTICE:

Do you recall a person in your early life who spoke to you in a way that made you believe you could not accomplish something? If so, can you think of ways this has manifested throughout your life?

Write your thoughts down in the space below. Finish with a short note (not to be delivered) to this person or persons telling them, in your own words, that they were wrong and how what they said or did made you feel.

Now think of a time when someone believed in you; perhaps not only encouraging you, but maybe even "expecting success". My mother had a phrase that exasperated me as a child, but as an adult I really began to understand it. Now I actually say it to myself! Whenever I thought a task was insurmountable, my mother would say, "That's no hill for a climber!" What Mom was saying to me in that very short phrase was, "You are a capable person, and this is not a challenge for someone with your ability."

Can you recall some ways people have encouraged and supported you along the way? Did their support help you to overcome self-doubt and accomplish a goal?

What did they say that encouraged you? Here again, you can write a short thank you note to the person or persons that come to mind. This may be a note that you actually wish to send.

Looking back to a time when you have accomplished a goal, how did you feel?

Write down your thoughts in the space below.

Now imagine that you are the grown up in your early life. What words would you use to encourage the "child-you" to achieve that goal? Can you think of times when you could use these words to reassure yourself in the present?

It is true that much of our "Self E" is established in childhood. However, we can experience our "Self E" waxing and waning throughout our lives as we encounter roadblocks and challenges along the way. Losing a job, searching for employment, scoring poorly on an exam, dealing with a failed relationship or agonizing over troubling family matters can all put our "Self E" to the test. I have found myself in situations like these more often than I care to comfortably admit. Looking back, I sometimes imagine myself as in "The Perils of Pauline"; the original damsel in distress. One episode featured a confluence of somewhat unrelated events from which I found myself, without a home, without a car, without a job, with my savings obliterated and just for good measure, a stalker. Just remembering that time makes my heart pound. But I always held on to my mother's reminder that I had the skills to climb out of that hole and make it over the hill. With her admonition as a lifeline, I took some deep breaths, gathered up my "Self E" and pulled myself out of the hole and over the hill.

The good news is that we can build on "Self E" throughout our lifetime as we realize that we can learn and grow and discover our talents in a variety of ways.

Sometimes we need encouragement from others. Sometimes seeing others who are like us succeed gives us the confidence to do the same. The BEST way to develop self efficacy is actually to have an objective or goal in mind and subsequently achieve that goal. But there is a catch: If we do try and fail, we have the potential to damage our self efficacy.

WHAT TO DO?

In the space below, write down the names of the people in your life who are encouraging and supportive to your dreams, goals and ambitions. Put these people on your "Self E" team. Consider letting them know you have put them on your *dream team* and that their assurance and support is valued and appreciated. You could even photograph yourself with them and have a "Self E"- selfie!

My Dream Team:

> As we go though the lessons in this book, you now know that you have a team of supporters ready to remind you that you are competent and capable of achieving your goals. When you come to a rough spot in the road (and we all do), and are feeling down, call someone on your dream team for a booster shot of encouragement.

PRACTICE:

Making a task list or "to-do" list is a good way to practice accomplishing small goals. On a separate sheet of paper, make a (short) list of 2 or 3 items that you need to get done today. This can be as simple as "water the plants" or "call my mom". Your self efficacy task is to do those things. The idea is to reinforce that you are capable of setting a goal and accomplishing the goal in a prescribed period of time. ***This practice is deliberately simple.*** We are practicing, deciding on a relevant goal, setting a time frame by which it must be accomplished, accomplishing the goal and (IMPORTANT) noticing how it feels to succeed and juice up our "Self E" for more challenging tasks down the road. When you have completed your list, give yourself a pat on the back! Perhaps you can begin to consider one or two larger, wellness-related goals. What might that look like for you?

THE THREE SELFS AND YOU

Remember that this book is for you and about you. It is an opportunity to discover how you can feel better and experience life more fully. You may be noticing that throughout the MIND section I have been asking you to get in touch with how you feel. It is especially important to really reflect on this. *How do you feel?*

Many years ago, I was a very busy working mother with two young children. I was trying to be supermom, super employee, super spouse, super homemaker. You can get a sense of it: Brownie Leader, soccer mom, church deacon, award winner, key player in a growing business and wife whose husband travelled for work. Oh! I was also trying to be a good daughter-in-law by accommodating my live-in mother-in-law. It was go, go, go until the end of the day, when I dropped into a chair to watch *Rugrats* with the kids and have a couple of glasses of wine. I thought I was fine. And though I was eating fairly well, exercising in moderation and getting my tasks accomplished, I was running on empty and, apparently, it showed. One day, a colleague from work pulled me aside and asked how I was doing. "What do you mean? I don't understand. I'm fine", I persisted. But then I admitted to myself, a little tired, a little sick. "Sick and tired." Impervious to my rebuff, my colleague pressed me, "How do you feel? "What do you *feel*?" The question stumped me. I honestly didn't know. I had been so busy, doing and achieving, ensuring that I accomplished all that I believed society expected of me, that I had completely lost touch with how I felt. How *did* I feel? I had no idea. But the question spurred me to go inward to figure it out, to continue to search for the feelings I desired most such as happiness, freedom, buoyancy and vigor. This was a turning point in my journey.

Recognizing and honoring our feelings is essential to our progression through the Three Selfs. Self esteem requires us to recognize and define our feelings. We are learning to feel good about ourselves. Self respect involves identifying our feelings when we are deserving of respect as well as realizing that, when we are not respectful to ourselves our feelings (self esteem) suffer as a consequence. "Self E" calls on us to acknowledge how we feel when we accomplish a goal. Having strong self efficacy helps us to finish the tasks we set out upon, to feel good about ourselves for having done so and to continue to take on new and worthwhile challenges.

How do *you feel*? This question changed my life. I believe it can change yours.

If you haven't done so already, it is time to ask yourself, what is your purpose in reading this book? Maybe you were just curious about the title. Perhaps you need something to put you to sleep at night. What do you anticipate will change as a result of taking the time to read this book and do the exercises? We are all unique individuals and have come to this place for different reasons. Perhaps you just want to feel better. What will it take for you to feel better? Better food choices? Moving more? Quiet time? Improved relationships? What does feeling better look like for you? What is your vision? Try to see it clearly in your mind. In his book "Quantum Healing", Deepak Chopra teaches us that what we think about today will be reflected in our bodies tomorrow. How we think about ourselves and the way in which we address our feelings literally changes us, both physically and emotionally. It affects how well we heal and our ability to thrive.

Now close your eyes for a moment and imagine how *you feel* when you have accomplished this vision of yourself.

In the space below, write down your vision and the feelings you experienced. Give yourself time to include as much detail as possible. Come back to this page frequently and check in. Maybe there will be something you want to change or to add. Go ahead - do it. You are in control of your future. What is it you desire?

The only person you are destined to become is the person you decide to be."

~ RALPH WALDO EMERSON

My Vision for Myself:

Now that you have established a vision for yourself and before turning the page to Chapter 2, take a moment to sit quietly with no distractions. Consider your vision as it contrasts your current state of wellness. Are you frequently sluggish or lethargic? Do you find yourself impatient or quick tempered? Do you feel heavy in your body, mind and spirit? If you could overlay your vision for yourself with your current state of wellness, would they match up? Let's take a look.

INTRODUCING THE WELLNESS RULER

The Wellness Ruler is a simple way to establish how you feel about your current state of wellness and compare the way you feel today with your "more-well" vision of yourself.

Looking at the Wellness Ruler, consider wellness as a spectrum ranging from 1-10, where 1 represents having little or no wellness qualities and 10 represents your ideal vision of wellness. Choose your own words to describe the points along the wellness spectrum.

Here are some ideas:

At the left side of the ruler you might use words such as:

Lethargic
Weary
Stressed
Overwhelmed
Powerless
Or choose a word that best describes this for you.

At the right side of the ruler you might use words such as:

Buoyant
Zestful
Vitality
Enthusiastic
Excited
Or choose a word that best describes this for you.

Some suggestions for points between 1 and 10 might be:
From 2-4:

Dull
Indifferent
Unmotivated

Weak
Lackluster

From 4-6

Accepting
Considering
Reasonable
Satisfactory

From 7-9

Energetic
Optimistic
Positive
Confident

On the Wellness Ruler below, make a point at which you find yourself now. On this point, write today's date and a word or two that describes how you feel at this point. If you can't come up with the exact descriptor for you, don't worry; if something new comes to you, you can always come back and write it down later. Next make a point that would describe the vision that you created for yourself. Are the two points different? What word(s) did you use to describe your vision-you?

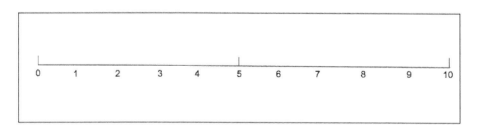

Now close your eyes and see yourself when you embody your vision and these descriptors.

Is your body weight different?

Can you move more freely?

Are your relationships better?

Is work easier and more productive?

Is the family happier?

What do **YOU** see? What do **YOU** feel?

Notes:

"Your vision will become clear only when you look into your heart. Who looks outside, dreams. Who looks inside, awakens."

~ CARL JUNG

THE THREE SELFS – ME, ME, WONDERFUL ME!

When my children were small we used to love Sesame Street. One of my favorite performances was Big Bird singing "Wonderful Me". (https://www.youtube.com/watch?v=pDGf_AEDDoY). "Wonderful Me" is a delightful expression of the Three Selfs. In just over two minutes we understand the sensation of feeling good about ourselves, of believing in our ability to accomplish our goals and respecting who we are and the character with which we show up in the world

In the context of wellness, we recognize that what Big Bird teaches, what we describe in the Three Selfs, is the foundation for genuine well-being. When we are feeling good about ourselves and have positive self esteem we are more likely to make constructive, healthful choices about food, activity and relationships. With self respect, we accept that we deserve to be treated with thoughtfulness, especially by ourselves to ourselves. And finally, "Self E" reminds us that we are capable of achieving our goals and ambitions. The Three Selfs literally are essential to our ability to succeed on our journey toward lifetime wellness. Take your time with this chapter, spend time with the practices and allow the Three Selfs to reveal themselves to you. If ever you find yourself feeling unsure about the Three Selfs, you can always revisit the practices in this chapter. And happily, Big Bird is just a click away as a reminder of Wonderful You!

"You yourself, as much as anybody in the entire universe, deserve your love and affection"

~ BUDDHA

2

Wellness Essential #2: Compassion

YOUR HIP POCKET HIPPOCRATES

"If your compassion does not include yourself, it is incomplete."

~ BUDDHA

How we experience our daily lives is directly associated with our ability to show compassion. What is compassion anyway? We can describe compassion as empathy, concern, kindness and care. We demonstrate compassion by taking time to sincerely understand feelings, being thoughtful, tending to needs and being gentle and benevolent. A beautiful illustration of how compassion can be reflected in our lives can be seen on the YouTube video, "The Power of True Kindness" (https://www. you tube.com/watch?v=W8OWKy_JBCc). If you can, take a moment now to view it.

Compassion is not just a modern, new-age, woo-woo concept in health. In fact, compassion is part of the Hippocratic Oath, a vow historically taken by most western medical doctors. Within the oath we find the phrase: *"I will remember that there is art to medicine as well as science, and that warmth, sympathy, and understanding may outweigh the surgeon's knife or the chemist's drug."* Research being conducted at Stanford University and the University of California, Berkeley is revealing that Hippocrates was really onto something. Science is proving that compassion for ourselves and others can enhance well-being, improve health and enrich relationships. Throughout our lives we have been taught to be kind and to be considerate of another's feelings. Certainly we have all felt sympathy for others in times of grief or despair. But most of us forget that we ourselves are deserving of compassion. Let's take a look at compassion and how it functions in our lives.

PRACTICE:

Think of people or instances in your life where you have had the opportunity to show compassion. What did you do? How did it make you feel? Write down your thoughts in the space below.

Often we are harder on ourselves than we would be on another person. We might berate or scold ourselves rather than show understanding and compassion.

Use the steps below to help you think of ways that you might show compassion for yourself.

Here are some ideas:

- Identify your feelings (Example: happy, sad, guilt, shame, fear, pride, jealousy, insecure etc.)
- Acknowledge your feelings. (Example:"Yes, I recognize that I am jealous of...")
- Accept yourself (your feelings, your life, your body) You are not a bad person because you are having these feelings. (Example: "I sometimes feel discouraged because my body isn't as buoyant as I would like it to be. Even so, I am blessed with good health and a positive outlook.")
- Create quiet time for rest and reflection. During your time of reflection, acknowledge that you are a good person and that you can make good decisions about your health and wellbeing. You have the power to make changes in your life. (Example: "I recognize that I could make better choices that would help improve my self esteem and self respect. I know I am capable of making better choices.")

Most of us need help remembering to be compassionate toward ourselves. Sometimes we may even need help accepting that we deserve compassion.

Let me be emphatically clear about this.

We ALL need compassion. **We ALL DESERVE compassion.**

One way to remember that we need and deserve to be compassionate with ourselves is with a brief statement, affirmation or mantra. In this case a nice short, easy to remember statement will do. Here are a few examples:

" I am loving and kind and deserving of compassion."

"I am worthy of respect and kindness."

"My feelings are important. I shall be tender with them."

"Loving myself does not take away from loving others."

"I deserve to treat myself with dignity and compassion."

You can adapt one of these to suit you or create your own. But do get started on the following activity right away:

- Create your compassion mantra
- Look in the mirror and say it to your reflection
- Repeat it with or without a mirror throughout the day

One of my favorite ways to incorporate a mantra into my day is to write my mantra down on a tiny piece of paper and keep it in my pocket. Each time I reach into my pocket and feel the piece of paper, I am reminded of my mantra.

Why talk about compassion in the context of whole person health and well-being?

Research tells us that cultivating compassion in our daily lives can help reduce pain, anxiety and blood pressure and help improve work performance, particularly in high stress jobs. It can also help improve our outlook on life and our ability to foster optimism and contentment.

As we pursue this idea of wellness, remember the wellness quote from the introduction, **"Wellness, it's the best in each of us..."**

Compassion is elemental to that which is the best in each of us. As we journey toward Lifetime Wellness, along the way we will constantly be faced with choices, undoubtedly make mistakes and have multiple set backs. Even with a strong sense of the Three Selfs, we still need compassion for ourselves not only to overcome challenges but to emerge stronger and wiser than we were before. The Dalai Lama teaches,

" *If you want others to be happy, practice compassion. If you want to be happy, practice compassion.*"

Can you remember a time when you have experienced a set back? We have all done things we regret, some things we regret more strongly than others. This could range from breaking a promise, to binge eating or drinking or to being disloyal. If we continually linger on the mistakes of the past, we will be led down a very sad and gloomy path indeed.

Remember Homer Simpson's famous quote, "*You can't keep blaming yourself. Just blame yourself once, and move on.*"

PRACTICE:

To learn how to follow Homer's advice, try this exercise:

Think of your most recent set back or regret. (I had one today when I snapped at my husband…)

1. Acknowledge what happened (just accept it for what it was – don't judge yourself). Example: "I snapped at my husband."
2. Give words to how this error made you feel. Example: regretful, embarrassed, angry, shameful, etc. "I regret losing my temper and snapping at him. I am ashamed of myself for behaving that way."
3. Look at the situation and try to understand, a) why or how it happened and b) how you could prevent this from happening again. Example: "I was in a hurry to get to my son's baseball game. I should have taken more time to communicate with my husband about how important getting to the game was to me and asked for his help and support."
4. Last step. Ask and answer: Why is it important to me to prevent this from happening again? Example: "My relationship with my husband is tremendously important to me. I don't want to hurt his feelings or our relationship due to my unnecessary impatience."
   Whether the slip-up is gorging on a bag of potato chips, pizza and ice cream, binging on alcohol, or snapping at your spouse or children, coming back to the four steps can help you forgive yourself and to make better choices in the future.

We are all human, and from time to time we all make mistakes and/or decisions we regret. Pursuing a healthier, happier life is a worthy, albeit demanding, goal. There will be times when we make regrettable choices. When blunders happen, come back to these four steps, always without judgment and always finishing with number four. This is an expression of compassion for yourself. It will help you reframe your experience, realizing that you have the power to improve your well-being and change your life.

RECAPPING COMPASSION

You have probably heard the adage that we can't fully love another until we love ourselves. The same is true of compassion. I believe we all want to be compassionate toward others. It is great to know that science is proving what Hippocrates professed thousands of years ago, that the warm-fuzzy feeling we have when we are compassionate is healing, both to ourselves and to others, on multiple levels. The piece we often miss is that we cannot give something we don't already have. Consequently, filling our own compassion tank gives us a reservoir that allows us to share with others. We cultivate compassion for ourselves when we accept that we are deserving of compassion, when we are gentle, kind and empathetic toward ourselves and when we acknowledge our mistakes and reason through our errors without berating ourselves. As we take the next steps on our journey, remember you can be the Hippocrates who heals your life. If you are having trouble expressing compassion toward yourself, come back to the work you did in this chapter and practice, practice, practice.

"When you have learned compassion for yourself, compassion for others is automatic."

~ HENEPOLA GUNARATANA

3

Wellness Essential #3: Mindful Awareness

"In the long run, we shape our lives, and we shape ourselves. The process never ends until we die. And the choices we make are ultimately our own responsibility."

~ ELEANOR ROOSEVELT

While there are many interpretations of mindful awareness, I define it in this way: *To keenly observe at all times what is happening with your environment, your thoughts and actions as well as the feelings and actions of those around you – without making judgments.* What a mouthful. It sounds daunting doesn't it? You are right. It can be! In our culture where multi-tasking reigns supreme, we are constantly busy doing so many things it is rare that we take the time to keenly observe anything. What does it mean to "keenly observe"? It means to look deeply into what is going on in our bodies, our minds and the world around us as well as how our words and actions effect others. Mindful awareness is all about the *choices* we make from moment to moment and the consequences of those choices. With all of that in mind, it also means that we do not cast our opinion or prejudice onto others. Yes, mindful awareness is quite a challenging endeavor. It may even be impracticable. But it is definitely worth the effort.

Most of us forget that we are actually making choices every moment of our lives. Many of our choices are so ingrained that they have become habits. We don't really need to think about them. We get out of bed. We brush our teeth. We get dressed. We have done these things for so long that we have forgotten that we are actually *choosing to do them.*

As mundane as these may seem they are all choices and are also, broadly, wellness behaviors. Staying in bed too long can wreak havoc with both our physical and mental well-being. Tooth brushing is essential to our physical and social health. Even the act of getting dressed and selecting what to wear reveals how we care for ourselves. While it is true that these behaviors are part of a humdrum routine, we have still *chosen* to make them part of our lives. Mindful awareness gives us the chance to shape our lives according to the multitude of choices we make.

Ram Das explained mindfulness with his beautifully simplistic reminder, *"Be here now."* Another way to describe mindful awareness is to be "present"; or put in a more common way, "Pay attention!"

Wait a minute….

What on earth does all of this have to do with "Wellness"?

When we begin to practice this level of keen awareness, our entire being benefits. Neuroscience research has shown that mindfulness training helps to:

- Reduce stress and anxiety
- Enhance immune function
- Reduce depression
- Improve relationships
- Improve sleep quality
- Reduce emotional reactivity
- Enhance creativity
- Decrease blood pressure
- Heighten empathy
- Improve problem solving capacity

Looking through this list it is easy to see how each of these physical responses corresponds to how we *feel* in our daily lives as well as how we cope with the challenges life sends our way.

The day I realized that I had lost touch with, *my feelings*, I understood that something had to change. I wasn't sure how to go about creating that change. I was already over committed with responsibilities and overextended emotionally and physically. How could I possibly add one more thing, particularly something that didn't appear to have tangible rewards and that took time away from all of my other duties? (Sound familiar?) But I knew I had to begin somewhere. That part of me that was lost was drifting further away and needed to be rescued. I began to explore books like, "Reflections on the Art of Living", by Joseph Campbell, and "Practicing the Presence" and the "Art of Meditation" by Joel Goldsmith. The teachings of these authors helped me to understand that because I had allowed myself to become so busy and so stressed, I needed to make time to reconnect with my feelings and the nature of the world around me. On weekdays, I would often pull the car over on the way to work, just to appreciate the sun coming over the mountains or the light reflecting on the landscape. Those few moments were the most I could give at the time. It was a beginning. Later, I found 30 - 45 minutes on weekends to take a walk, alone. As I walked into my nature retreat and took in the beauty of my surroundings, bit-by bit, day-to-day stress and concern dropped along the trail behind me. I would find a beautiful serene spot to sit, enjoy nature and clear my mind. On the walk home, the bits I had left on the trail were gone. My mind was clear. I felt renewed.

If this kind of thing is new for you, it's best to start simply.

PRACTICE

Lets take a quick (and easy) practice moment. Really – carve out a moment or two to focus on just this practice.

Look outside. What is the weather like? Is it sunny and warm; cold and icy? Maybe it is dark and cloudy or a starry night. Is the moon out? Is the wind blowing? How hard? Can you see trees moving in the wind? What do you hear? Wind blowing, children playing, dogs barking? Are there people outside? How are they interacting with the weather or with each other? Can you tell if they are happy? Hurried? Emotionless?

Maybe you can go outside. How does the air feel against your skin? How does it smell?

Take in as many observations as you can and integrate them into your bodymind. Actually *"sense them".*

Congratulations! You have just taken a moment to be present, to be fully aware, utilizing all of the faculties at your disposal. Experiencing nature is a lovely and simple way to begin taking more and more steps toward paying attention all of the time.

The idea of Wellness Essential #3 is to bring this level of awareness to everything in your daily life. It may seem overwhelming at first. Just remember, this is a journey. It begins with small steps. Thich Nhat Hahn beautifully reminds us to be mindful; *"Walk as if you are kissing the Earth with your feet."*

PRACTICE:

Over the next few days, find a moment (at least one) in your day to STOP, breathe and observe nature. Do your best to experience what you observe. See it, feel it, smell it, commune with it, embrace it. Each time you do this – notice how you feel before and also after. Note: Sometimes we may feel apprehensive about noticing and becoming aware of feelings. In those situations pausing to do this exercise may feel uncomfortable. It may help to go back to the Three Selfs and consider how you feel in a variety of situations. When you feel you are ready, return here and try again. Remember - baby steps.

This practice is about more than just experiencing nature. Our goal is to create more and more moments of awareness and connect them together throughout the day like connecting points of interest on your journey, or creating a string of pearls. As we begin to become more mindfully aware, we also begin to notice more and more instances when we have the power to decide how we wish to experience our lives.

When we practice mindful awareness on a regular basis, we are actually remodeling our brains. With any consistent thought or behavior pattern, our brains undergo an architectural transformation. Throughout our lives, our experiences, thoughts, emotions and behaviors have created a sort of structure in our brains, as though we have built a home for them. Most of us feel quite comfortable in this home, indeed! So it might be difficult to imagine what our remodeled home will look like. We might need to tear down a few walls, add some support beams, change a few colors and add windows and light. Appealing as this sounds, it will take patience, time, effort and *consistent* work. Also, change of this nature can require that we get dirty and dusty as we tear down the old and prepare for the new. Along with this we will undoubtedly have to discard some things that we have become attached to, and that can sometimes feel like a loss. This remodel will likely feel uncomfortable at times, but the end result will be the home of our dreams!

This is absolutely the case with our brains. We begin life with bright and open hearts and minds. But many of us experience a rough road or a terrible crisis that we get through but choose not to look at or think about. We may have suffered the trauma of abuse or war or death of a loved one. Experiences such as these can cause us to "build walls" in our minds. These walls cause us to adopt behavior patterns that enable us to maneuver around without even noticing they exist.

Sometimes when these things happen, we cover up the windows of our minds to prevent the view. Over time, we simply learn to adapt to this dark, confining mental infrastructure. Often the hurt is so deep or distant, we even forget what caused us to build our structure this way in the first place. What we have is what we are familiar with and that familiarity can provide a distorted sense of comfort.

As we become more mindful and aware, we begin to perceive the walls we have built and the darkness we have become accustomed to. Mindful awareness is like a loving demolition crew that, using the tools of new thought patterns, allows us to begin bringing down the walls, opening the blocked views and remodeling the structures we have constructed in our brains. We begin to uncover the reasons we put up those walls and shut out the view. We begin to see more clearly. This can be hard work and it can sometimes be painful. But if we have courage, knowing that we are creating a better space, and the persistence to work at it daily, eventually we will have a sparkling new, more resilient, beautiful, light-filled space that allows consciousness to flow freely and confidently.

"Your true home is in the here and the now."

~ THÍCH NHÂT HẠNH

WHAT PREVENTS US FROM BEING MINDFULLY AWARE? DISTRACTION AND JUDGMENT

Jon Kabat-Zinn describes mindfulness as "suspension from distraction". I love that description because, in our culture, distractions are practically ceaseless. We see televisions on in restaurants and doctors' offices, solicitors have hijacked our phones and email accounts, everyone it seems wants to alert us to something they believe to be important regardless of the time of day or night. What does it mean to suspend distraction? Very simply, it is just taking a time out. Another way to approach the idea of suspending distraction is to establish priorities for what is important to us at any given moment and to stay true to those priorities.

The window of my studio looks out over a beautiful fountain that, in the summer, is surrounded by beautiful flowers, butterflies and small children enamored with it all. Throughout the summer, parents and their children pass by. The kids excitedly call out to their grown-ups, "Mommy look, look!" "Daddy, watch this!" Too often the grown-ups are distracted by a text, phone call or facebook. The young ones eventually give up. It makes me feel sad when I see they get the message; they are not the priority at the moment.

I am certain that you can think of everyday distractions that cause you to get sidetracked from what you are doing or struggle to maintain concentration because of some nagging and persistent interruption.

ALL HAIL KING MULTI-TASK

From the everyday situations such as cooking dinner and talking on the phone, to those with negative consequences such as texting and driving, we live in an age where multi-tasking is king. We believe our gadgets and devices keep us plugged in, tuned in and connected. The fact is, we are less "connected" than ever before.

It is true that many of these tools help keep us safe, stay in touch with loved ones and have revolutionized business and industry. The irony is that the very things that have the ability to keep us engaged, focused and make life easier have become distractions that keep us disconnected and bleary. While many of us take pride in our ability to multi-task and take advantage of all the gadgets that allow us to do so, the truth is that whenever we are multitasking we are not fully present or aware in any given situation. While our brains are the most miraculous computers in the world, they actually suffer when we obsessively multi-task. Research carried out at the University of London revealed that while simple multi-tasking, such as receiving phone calls or emails during a meeting or problem solving tasks, participants in the study experienced a significant drop in IQ. This drop in IQ during multitasking has since been compared to functioning at the level of an 8 year old. According to a report by the BBC, the corresponding drop in IQ that occurs with multi-tasking is more than twice that found in studies looking at brain function impairment and marijuana.

When multi-tasking, our brains cannot effectively complete one task and we don't shift from one task to another as well as if we were focused on one thing at a time. Additionally, because we have become so attuned to listening for the magic chime of incoming messages, news updates or favorite songs, our brains remain on high alert, which keeps us in a state of constant mental stress. Over time we find ourselves actually dependent on the distractions. A.K.A. *Addicted.*

The word *addicted* may feel emotionally charged or too strong to be used in conjunction with our precious, prized electronic paraphernalia. However, the stimuli of all the bells and beeps along with the instant satisfaction associated with receiving and responding to these alerts, actually delivers a pleasure rush due to the brain, not unlike certain drugs. It is kind of mind-boggling to consider that most of us have a gadget of some sort that we feel compelled to respond to when it beckons. If the majority of us find ourselves in these multi-tasking situations throughout the day, during which we may have a drop in our functional IQ, what does that say about how our society is functioning as a whole?

While more and more research is being done in this area, one thing is for certain. When we are multi-tasking we are not fully present in any singular endeavor. What this means to us and our well-being is that when we are consumed with multi-tasking we make poorer choices, our work may not reflect our true brilliance and our relationships suffer because we are not able to listen or communicate clearly and effectively.

JUDGMENT & MINDFUL AWARENESS

> *"If you judge a book by its cover, you might miss out on an amazing story."*
>
> *~ UNKNOWN*

We have come a long way in our conversation about mindful awareness. As a reminder, our definition of the mindful awareness wellness essential is: *To keenly observe what is happening with your environment, your thoughts and actions as well as the feelings and actions of those around you at all times – without making judgments.*

…Without making judgments. As we begin to be more aware of our environment and surroundings it is inevitable that we will observe situations that will be off-putting, annoying, or maybe even infuriating. Our reactions to these situations are often the result of how we judge the situation or person. To practice mindful awareness as we discuss it in this book, we must truly grasp the notion of observing without judging.

THE (KNEE) JERK

Too often in our culture we want to label a person or a situation. Here is how easily it happens. Someone cuts us off in traffic, or blocks the aisle at the grocery store, or uses a sharp tone of voice over the phone, or refuses to be helpful. We observe these actions and, typically, immediately make a judgment that goes something like this; "That person is a reckless so-in-so (jerk) !" "She is so inconsiderate and self-involved (what a "jerk")!" "He is such a @#&*(jerk)!" "She is a stupid _____ (jerk)" "What an idiot!" These kinds of comments are so reflexive. They are "knee-jerk" reactions and are so common that we don't even realize we are actually judging. It can be as simple as judging others based on the type of clothes they wear, their jewelry (piercings), body type or tattoos, to judging people for their political or religious affiliations.

Admit it. We make knee-jerk judgments all the time. By placing labels on people rather than the actions we observe, we are judging them.

What we want to strive for instead is to observe the situation and change our language. By learning to change our words and observations, eventually we can change our minds. The difference might sound something like this, "That person is really driving recklessly. That is a really dangerous thing to do!" "That person's cart is blocking the aisle. It is such an inconvenience to have to go around", "He was really abrupt with me on the phone." "I don't understand why she was so unhelpful."

SO WHAT IF I JUDGE? WHAT DOES THAT HAVE TO DO WITH MY HEALTH?

When we are judging others, we can often experience unhealthy emotions such as anxiety, anger, irritation and stress. Over time (and remember we tend to judge constantly) all of these emotions carry with them physiological responses, which include: depressed immune function, digestive troubles, increased weight, increased blood pressure, depression, anxiety and more. Giving up judgment requires that we notice when we engage in judging and make a mindful decision to let it go. You will find that you will begin to feel better right away. This *feel better sensation* will impact your health immediately as well as long term.

JUDGE ME JUDGE YOU

Another component to judging others has to do with placing our own undesirable qualities, fears or feelings onto another person or situation. You have probably heard the admonition, *when you point a finger at someone else, three are pointing back at you.* Some examples of this type of judging include labeling people as arrogant, untrustworthy, selfish, undisciplined or lazy. It can be rather uncomfortable to look at this, but it is important to our journey, so let's take a moment to go through it.

PRACTICE

Think of someone who annoys you or whom you simply don't care for. Ask yourself what it is about this person that bothers you. Listen to what you are telling yourself. (Is that person a show-off, ignorant, grumpy, whiny, controlling, etc.) Now (here's the hard part) apply the three-finger test.

Finger #1 Can you identify characteristics in yourself that are similar? (Example: I can be somewhat self-involved.)

Finger #2 Can you remember a time when you may have acted the same way? (Example: I noticed that I got impatient and annoyed when Josie waited until the last minute to cancel our appointment because she was sick.)

Finger #3 How do you think other people perceive you when you do this? (Example: When I lose patience and become annoyed at this type of thing, I must seem selfish and unfeeling.)

This first three-finger test opens a window that allows us to see our own issues honestly and perhaps more clearly. Once we are able to view our own behaviors objectively, we can try taking the next steps toward lessening our tendency to judge and healing our inner selves.

One way to do this is to use our propensity to fix others to help fix ourselves. Just as we can easily identify what annoys us about other people, we can also easily come up with ideas about what that person could (should) do to be more to our liking. The same advice we would offer others, we can apply to ourselves. With this in mind, just as we turned the three fingers toward ourselves above, let's try it again.

Finger #1 I recognize that there is a part of me who acts like this in certain situations. (Example: Yes, I can be selfish and unfeeling)

Finger #2 I remember behaving this way when........ (Example: I act this way when I feel others are inconsiderate.)

Finger #3 The next time I find myself faced with this situation, I will be mindful and make the choice to change my behavior. (Example: I will try to catch myself when these feelings come up and try to be more understanding of the other person's situation.)

When you are able to recognize this aspect of judgment and do the three finger exercise, you are able to recognize characteristics in yourself that you find undesirable in others. You free yourself of the negative emotions and physiological damage associated with judging. You can then begin to better understand yourself and to take another step toward well-being and happiness.

Finally, in our discussion on judgment (or avoiding judgment) we need to talk about attachment. Attachment, in the framework of our conversation, can be driven by fear and deals with being emotionally attached to a situation. When we are attached to a situation, it is difficult to see past how the situation affects us personally. Often, when we find ourselves in a situation that causes a knee-jerk judgment, we are reacting to a deeper attachment. Maybe someone's actions have caused us to fear for our safety or well-being, maybe we feel threatened, offended or simply annoyed. This is the time to make two more choices:

First, as Don Miguel Ruiz simply reminds us in "The Four Agreements", **"Don't take it personally."** In other words, the things people do or say come from their own issues, problems or concerns. Having a disapproving reaction to the behaviors of others basically puts their "stuff" in your toy box. It is not yours. Don't make it yours.

Second, instead of putting your own "stuff' onto someone else, recognize that the person or situation – the object of your judgment - may have problems that you are not aware of. That reckless driver? Maybe a loved one was rushed to the hospital and she is racing to get there to be by his side. The person who was abrupt on the phone? Maybe he was just fired from that job. The person whose cart is blocking the aisle? Maybe she has a physical or mental impairment that causes confusion or trouble processing. The person who spoke in a sharp tone? Maybe she is being abused at home. We can never know. But we can choose not to attach to the situation, choose not to get angry or upset, and rather than labeling or judging, try to project understanding or forgiveness.

"Be kind, for everyone you meet is fighting a hard battle."

~ PLATO

LOOKING BACK AT MINDFUL AWARENESS

As we come to the close of our discussion on mindful awareness, remember that as difficult and multifaceted as it may seem, mindful awareness is really about merely trying. We are trying to be aware of our thoughts, feelings and actions. We are trying to notice the world around us, endeavoring to pause and detach from our hasty reactions and, instead, to act with empathy and kindness. The change begins in the *attempt* to stop and notice, to recognize or re-think situations and opinions. Noticing that you are noticing is a huge accomplishment.

Just keep trying. Appreciate beauty in all its forms. Appreciate the struggles each of us face in our lives that may cause us to act or react in various ways. And lastly, don't forget to appreciate yourself for making the effort to be mindfully aware.

> *"Mindfulness is about being fully awake in our lives. It is about perceiving the exquisite vividness of each moment. We also gain immediate access to our own powerful inner resources for insight, transformation, and healing."*
>
> ~ *JON KABAT-ZINN*

MIND REVISITED

Early on in our conversation I shared with you the Three Essentials of Wellness. I told you that once you have these Essentials in your grasp, making your journey toward lifetime wellness would be simply a matter of choices. Generally, when we decide we want to embark on a healthier lifestyle, we tend to focus on a physical and nutritional regimen. We just want someone to tell us what "to do" and what "to eat", and we promise ourselves and others that we can and will follow the program. Essentially, we think we must give up our ability to choose for ourselves. But we must ALWAYS make a choice. In the case of a diet and exercise regimen, the choice most of us make is to give up. The fact is that without the foundation of the Three Essentials, no program will work.

This is not a "quick-fix" program. Living a model of wellness requires that we make healthful choices, on-going, everyday for the rest of our lives. The ability to make good choices comes from the basics of Self Esteem, Self Respect, and "Self E". Often times these are difficult choices to make. As we undertake the commitment to choosing a wellness lifestyle, compassion supports us by providing a kind and gentle nudge that enables us to begin healing at a deep emotional level and tenderly shepherding us to stay the course. Finally, cultivating Mindful Awareness enables us to get in touch with our feelings and notice how we are influenced by the way we interact with our environment. Having this awareness gives us the ability to harness unhealthy behaviors and emotions and transform our well-being at the cellular level.

With the Three Essentials, we are beginning to see that wellness is not really as much a state of being as it is an approach to living. We see that the activity of our minds is intricately related to our physical health. As we begin to adjust our mindset, our bodies will begin to feel lighter and more receptive to change.

Changing your mind will change your body and change your world.

Now that we have the Three Essentials in our grasp, we can begin our conversation about the more tangible, physical components of wellness.

"The sound body is the product of the sound mind."

~ GEORGE BERNARD SHAW

Section 2

Body

"We are beautiful because we are sons and daughters of God, not because we look a certain way."

~ KATE WICKER

Take a deep breath. Close your eyes and think about your body. What comes to mind?

Do you feel the mechanical miracle of the heart and lungs pumping away, continually supplying your cells with oxygen and nourishment? Do you see the spark of the billions of electrical impulses that allow for thoughts, emotions and movement? Can you sense the fluidity of chemical processes that produce energy and metabolism?

Probably not.

When we think about our bodies, we tend to bypass the ongoing internal second by second miracles and, instead, dwell on external images and perceptions; perhaps the reflection that stared back at us the last time we tried on a swimsuit or how we compare to others we have seen at the gym. Intellectually, we can appreciate the miraculous intricacies of the human body. But emotionally we tend to get stuck on our body image, our personal perception of how we think we look. The unfortunate companion to body image is our old friend judgment. Body image and judgment inevitably tend to join hands and become severe taskmasters. They can make talking about our bodies in an honest and compassionate way very uncomfortable and sometimes even painful.

Everywhere we turn we are flooded with images of "beautiful" bodies in magazines, tabloids, billboards and television. The media uses these images to sell product of course, but the way in which it is done creates stereotypes and leads us to make judgments about ourselves and others based on body image. These judgments can range from good/bad, to smart/stupid, to attractive/ugly to young/old. I think it is disgraceful that some person in advertising, casting or editing has the ability to define what is beautiful or healthy and has the capacity to shape our own self-worth as well as how others perceive us and judge us! Worse than that is the fact that through the miracle of editing, these perfect models and superstar images are not even real. They have been edited and photo-shopped to fit some third party's idea of beauty. As a result, our body image suffers because we are judging ourselves against a false standard. When we do this, how can we ever be good enough?

We have also received messages about body image from people who are close to us such as our parents, schoolmates or colleagues. Maybe someone made a comment about body types that felt as though it was directed at us. Maybe someone was deliberately cruel. Maybe there was unspoken bias in the home or the workplace.

These things are not only unkind, but they are also detrimental to our ability to develop a positive sense of self and to discover the power we have to realize, as our wellness definition reminds us, **"That which is the best in each of us."** It is time to let go of these judgments and beliefs about our bodies. We must not allow someone or something outside of ourselves to determine our self-worth.

BODY (IMAGE) BUILDING

Developing positive body image requires tending to our self esteem and self respect. It necessitates that we cultivate compassion for ourselves and for others, particularly with regard to body type. Ultimately, we must be mindfully aware of our tendency to judge others based on appearance lest we also feel judged.

PRACTICE:

Now it is time, once again, to take a personal inventory. Earlier, we did a practice with the Wellness Ruler. Let's do it again. This time, as you select your descriptive words and select your personal point on the ruler, try to integrate all that we have talked about thus far, the Three Selfs, Compassion, Mindful Awareness, and our brief discussion on the body and body image. It might help to think about the Wellness Ruler like a scale on your personal roadmap to wellness. If possible, use words similar to those you selected previously. If you are struggling to remember the words you used, flip back to your Wellness Ruler practice in the Three Selfs. Here are some of the words I suggested earlier if you need a mental nudge. Remember that as you consider your descriptors and select your point on the ruler that you are taking into account how your body feels and your body image.

At the left side of the ruler you might use words such as:

Lethargic

Weary

Stressed

Overwhelmed

Powerless

Or choose a word that best describes this for you.

At the right side of the ruler you might use words such as:

Buoyant

Zestful

Vitality

Enthusiastic

Excited

Or choose a word that best describes this for you.

Some suggestions for points between 1 and 10 might be:

From 2-4:

Dull
Indifferent
Unmotivated
Weak
Lackluster

From 4-6

Accepting
Considering
Reasonable
Satisfactory

From 7-9

Energetic
Optimistic
Positive
Confident

The object of this practice is to begin to recognize that how we feel about our bodies affects how we feel overall. Also, how we feel overall is interrelated with our sense of physical health and well-being. On the Wellness Ruler below, take into consideration the following:

- How you are feeling physically,
- The Three Essentials of Wellness and
- Your personal body image

Put a mark on the ruler with today's date that indicates how you are feeling today. As you continue on your path toward Lifetime Wellness, you can check in with the ruler to see how far you have come.

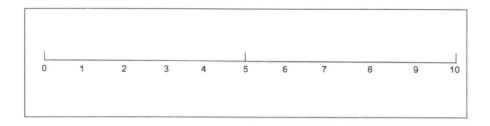

If you did not mark "10", take a moment to revisit your vision from chapter one and consider what you would need to do to move further right on the Wellness Ruler.

Choose better food? Move more? Improve your relationship with yourself and others?

This is also a time to recall that we are on a journey toward a lifetime of wellness. Along the way, we want to keep the right side of the Wellness Ruler in mind. The right side of the ruler represents your vision of a healthy, happy you. Keeping this in mind, we have a clearer idea of our purpose and can make better day-to-day choices that enhance our self respect and self efficacy. From time to time, there will be situations that arise when we do not or are not able to make the best choice toward buoyant health and well-being, whether it's overindulging at Thanksgiving, falling off the movement plan, finishing the entire pizza or having that extra glass of wine. These are the times to remember the practice we did in the Compassion chapter. We must be compassionate with ourselves, acknowledge we could have made a better choice and determine our strategy for making a better choice next time.

Remember, this is a journey that will take us through the rest of our lives. As with all journeys it begins with the first step. Now that you have taken a candid, yet compassionate, inventory of where you are right now and where you would like to go, let's begin to look at steps you can take now that will lead you in the direction of your life of wellness.

IT'S YOUR BODY. OWN IT!

"If you own this story you get to write the ending."

~ BRENÉ BROWN

While the "Three Essentials" (Three Selfs, Compassion and Mindful Awareness) are critical to our success in making decisions that lead us along the path of lifetime wellness, clearly optimal health and well-being don't just magically appear. Even if we have healthy self esteem, strong self respect and a high level of self efficacy, ultimately we still have to *decide we are ready* to change. In order for our desired change to occur, we have to feel good about that decision, care enough about ourselves to make change and have the confidence to know WE CAN DO IT!

Unfortunately, because there is such a glut of information about health and wellness everywhere we turn, trying to make sense of it all feels complicated, confusing and overwhelming. How can anyone know what is best?

GOOD NEWS!

This is the part where we take all the confusing clutter of information and boil it down into simple, logical concepts and learn the foundation for making better choices that will help you feel better every step of the way on your road to wellness. These choices are fundamentally yours. You OWN them. When you OWN something you take responsibility for it and have control over it. You *care* for it. So our easy to remember acronym to boil down your wellness choices is OWN; Oxygen, Water and Nourishment. Below we have a quick overview of OWN. As we venture further into our Body section will be talking about each one of these in wonderfully interesting detail.

O – Oxygen. Breathe. Sounds pretty simple doesn't it? Obviously we must have oxygen to survive. Coming up we will be talking more about some of the most important things we can do to deliver clean, life sustaining oxygen to every cell in our bodies. But for now, simply relax into a nice, long, slow deep breath and notice how refreshing and soothing something so simple can be!

W – Water. Pure water, and plenty of it. Of course we must have water to survive as well. Our adult bodies are roughly 55-70% water. It is essential to all of our organs and tissues – even bones! Water helps every system in our bodies to work better. It helps cushion our joints, soften our skin and reduce wrinkling. Water supports healthy brain and spinal fluid functions, is critical for a healthy heart, lungs and circulatory system and helps to deliver nutrients to our cells and to get rid of waste. We are fortunate to live in a country where clean drinking water is readily available and, basically, free!

Does all of this make you thirsty? Maybe a chilled glass of water with a slice of cucumber would be refreshing, or try a soothing cup of warm water with a lemon wedge.

N – Nourishment. Unfortunately, words like diet and nutrition have been used to describe rigid, restrictive eating plans or stern warnings or recommendations about what we can and cannot eat. The words diet and nutrition alone have begun to feel oppressive and difficult. But the "N" in our OWN should instead conjure up inviting, comforting images of nurturing and nourishment. It is really as simple as giving and receiving; giving your cells what they *need* and, in receiving what they need, your cells give back with bright, happy functioning that wards off disease and fatigue and illuminates your being from the inside out. Nourish your body from the inside out to reveal your "inner glow."

PRACTICE

Take a moment to look through a magazine that offers healthy recipes. Find a photo of a specific food or meal that you might be interested in exploring. Cut out the photo and save it. Write down a few words about why you selected this food to nourish your body and save it with your photo. Does looking at the photo and reading the words you selected produce any kind of change in how you feel? Do you feel more positive about your health just by seeing the photo and reading your words? It can happen! Imagine how great you will feel when you actually incorporate healthy food choices along your wellness journey.

Thus far we have talked a lot about the fact that in order to improve our health we must be aware that we have important decisions to make and that those choices need to be made with mindful awareness. We have begun to explore the relationship between mind and body and how our thoughts affect our health and well-being.

Realizing that all of the information we see and hear about exercise and diet can be conflicting, frustrating, overwhelming, and even paralyzing, we are bravely moving forward by simplifying and categorizing the areas in which we will need to make choices by using our easy acronym OWN.

Now let's take some time to break each one down in detail and give you a chance to practice and record the choices you will make as you continue along your journey.

"Go confidently in the direction of your dreams! Live the life you've imagined."

~ HENRY DAVID THOREAU

4

O is for Oxygen.

"Breathing is the first act of life. Our very life depends on it. Millions have never learned to master the art of correct breathing...."
"Therefore above all, learn to breathe correctly."

~ *JOSEPH HUBERTUS PILATES*

Breathing. Seems like a simple concept. We do it all day everyday without thinking. Our magical autonomic nervous system keeps air moving in and out throughout our lives. So why is something that occurs without any thought to it whatsoever part of our wellness plan? Our breath is more to our essential wellness than simply the exchange of oxygen and carbon dioxide. The way we breathe can influence wellness in many ways including our emotional and mental health, as well as posture, self image and even digestion.

To understand this relationship more fully, it might help to picture the movement of the diaphragm (the muscle that moves air in and out of the lungs) like ocean waves. When the ocean is calm, the waves are peaceful and soothing. Just thinking about it is calming. On the other hand, waves on a stormy sea are dark, churning, chaotic and tumultuous. Can you imagine what your body feels like when the diaphragm is pulling and pushing air in and out like waves in a storm? Tense, uptight, anxious, upset or nauseous come to mind.

The cause of these stormy episodes is an upset in the delicate balance between our breath and our brain. Interestingly, our emotions can affect our breath and our breath can affect our emotions. They are as intricately connected as the cogs in a timepiece (remember the old pocket watch?). When one spring is over wound the entire piece will coil up as well. But what is winding us up? For most of us, it is one pervasive, relentless culprit.

STRESS.

Let's take a moment to talk about stress and tension and overall heath and well-being. Here we are not talking about the good kind of stress that we experience with exercise for example. We are talking about the kind of stress that seems never ending; the stress that sends you into a panic or a tizzy or downright anger. You know what I mean; sick kids, pressures at work, car breaks down, house guests, frozen computer, spilled milk, traffic jams, late to work; the list is endless. Maybe you have heard the old saying, "If its not one thing, it's half-a-dozen!" Over a period of time, this chronic, uncontrolled stress – the bad kind of stress - wreaks havoc with the precious balance that our bodies strive so diligently to maintain. Just like a circus performer on a high wire, when we lose our balance bad things happen. As a result, almost every disease, ranging from the common cold to heart disease, cancer and even autoimmune disease is rooted in chronic stress.

At the first sign of stress, our amazing autonomic nervous systems begin a cascade of hormonal responses. These responses are a carry-over from our primitive days and their purpose is to provide alertness and stamina in the face of an emergency. This is what is known as the "fight or flight" response. As a result, our breath can become shallow and more rapid. When this happens, our muscles tense and our heart rate goes up. This can cause increased anxiety and muscle tension that shows up as headaches, neck pain and backaches. Because we often deal with multiple types of "bad stress" most days of the week, we never fully recover from each stress episode before another one hits. When we don't take the time to regain control of stress or manage the stress we are experiencing, our body's protective responses and systems begin to break down and the disease process begins to take hold.

This is where the O comes in. Most stress reduction techniques involve how we manage our breath. The beauty of the breath is that it is one function that we can control relatively easily. The power of the breath and various methods of breath control have been written about extensively for thousands of years, particularly in the Yogic traditions.

"I take refuge in breath, for verily breath is everything here that has come to be, whatsoever there is."

~ CHANDOGYA UPANISAD (3.15.4), BETWEEN THE 8TH AND THE 7TH CENTURY BCE. (23)

More recently, health experts in medicine, neuroscience and psychology have been studying various breathing techniques and their effects on stress reduction and long term health. Along with the many ways attention to your breath can aid in stress reduction to improve health, healthy breathing is also associated with improved digestion, enhanced delivery of nutrients to the cells and removal of waste, as well as decreased low back pain, mobility and circulation. The list goes on. But one fun fact about breath: when researchers asked the question, what actually happens to fat when we lose fat weight, the answer they discovered? We remove most of it through our breath!

Here are three quick and easy tips for adding more O to your daily life:

1. You have heard the phrase, "Before you get angry, count to 10." Rather than just counting to 10, count 10 breaths. Nice, long, slow breaths. Instead of experiencing a negative response to the stress or anger, your breath will help produce relaxation and inner calm. Your body will thank you for all the positive effects of breath.

2. Yawn. That's right! A host of research has been done on yawning. Our bodies and brains *need* to yawn and really benefit from yawning. In their book, "How God Changes Your Brain," authors Newberg and Waldman list a dozen reasons to yawn including that it stimulates concentration, reduces stress, broadens consciousness and enhances pleasure. In our society, yawning in public is considered rude or a sign of boredom. As a result, we have been conditioned not to yawn. So it may take some practice to allow yourself to yawn, but the rewards are worth it. Give it a try!

3. Talk less, listen more. What does this have to do with breathing? When we are talking, we are exhaling. Have you ever tried to speak during an inhale? People who need to do a lot of speaking for a living or folks who are simply chatterboxes, tend to breathe more shallowly, taking only sips of air in

between phrases. Because they spend so much time "exhaling", their bodies are not deriving much benefit from inhaling. To reap the benefits of O, we need to deepen our breath, allow time for the diaphragm to contract and relax, and give our cells the opportunity to receive oxygen and rid our bodies of waste.

"If we were supposed to talk more than we listen, we would have two tongues and one ear."

~ MARK TWAIN

Just For Fun (and health of course!)
Try this breathing exercise. This is especially fun to do with small children and they will also reap the benefits of simply breathing.

Lie in a comfortable place on your back, preferably something not too soft. A firm bed, sofa, carpeted floor or exercise mat will do. If you are doing this with a child and have a child's bath toy, that would be great! A small boat or ducky works well. Breathing solo? How about a small bag of rice or beans? Even your imagination will do nicely.

Begin by taking a few moments to relax your body into the surface you are lying on. If you have your toy or bag of rice you can place it on your belly, just below your belly button. Relax your jaw, your neck, your hands and your pelvis. How take your attention to your breath. Notice how the breath flows in and out, without effort. Just take a moment to notice your relaxed breath. Imagine your low belly is the ocean or a large body of water, and your boat or ducky is floating along on the waves.

Experience the waves of your belling rising and falling. Now deepen your exhale and feel your boat "sinking" into your belly. Your inhales bring the boat back to the crest of the wave. As your exhales deepen, so do the deep muscles of your abdomen.

Follow this breath pattern several times. Finally, allow the breath to soften once again, letting your boat to gently rise and fall on the calmer waters.

You have just taken a few moments to connect with your breath, to allow your diaphragm to fully expand and contract and to deliver essential oxygen to your tissues. Enjoy taking moments like these to nurture your entire body.

THE MOST FABULOUS AND INDESPENSIBLE WAY TO GET MORE O...
Start a MOVEMENT

> *"Life is activity, and when we stop being active we turn away from the new-ness of life."*

> *~ ERNEST HOLMES*

Thus far we have focused on Oxygen and our breath as it relates to stress management and other vital health benefits. But our conversation would not be complete if we did not discuss O as it relates to E. Exercise. I hesitate to use the word exercise because for many people it has a negative connotation. Often, when we think of exercise, other E words come to mind: exertion, exhaustion, effort. The E-word may also conjure up other unpleasant thoughts such as: hard, sweaty, time-consuming, grueling or even painful. Why put myself through that when my couch is such a welcoming companion?

I propose we forget about exercise. Instead, let's focus on simply moving, *mindfully*. Moving mindfully involves taking the Three Essentials (3 Selfs, Compasssion and Mindful Awareness) into your movement practice. Ahh. Mindful Movement. The words alone sound so much more gentle, forgiving and reasonable. They make you *want* to breathe. (Maybe a sigh of relief...right?)

Have you ever watched babies as they explore movement? Moving brings them joy. They giggle and laugh. They are delighted by the simple exploration of how their bodies can move.

Our bodies are actually designed to move. I know it may not feel like it at times, but everything about the way our bodies function is enhanced and flourishes with movement. The brain becomes keener. Organs are more efficient. Circulation improves. Digestion improves. Muscles and joints function better. The skeletal system is activated. Mood is lifted. Everything. Every system and function all the way down to each and every one of our billions of individual cells is improved with movement. Even our essence, our deep identifying nature, is brightened with movement.

I believe that through the course of our lives, for whatever reason, we lose the joy of movement. It becomes a chore, perhaps sheer drudgery. For some of us movement may feel like punishment. For some, it may have actually been used as punishment.

When we have had unpleasant experiences with exercise and movement, it is understandably a real challenge to overcome our reluctance to try it again. However, we need to rethink our perception of movement. We need to rediscover the joy that each of us had as babies as we explore what our bodies can do and achieve.

PRACTICE

Take a moment now to sit quietly and remember a time when simply moving gave you pleasure or enjoyment. Was there a time as a small child? Maybe experiencing a playground, or playing with family, friends or a pet? Try to recall the sensation of delight. What were you experiencing in your body and soul? In the space below, write down your memory. Try to find at least three positive words to describe how you felt.

Hold on to those feelings while we talk more about movement.

In recent years much research has been done to look at the health risks associated with a lot of sitting and the importance of simple movements throughout the day to prevent those health issues. As it turns out, ALL movement is meaningful. We know that very simple, basic actions such as standing, pacing, stretching and even toe tapping all have positive effects on our health and well-being, even for folks who do the "E-word" regularly. Our bodies actually NEED to get up and move around **frequently**. That part seems reasonably doable - right? If you are in a job or doing work at home that requires you to sit for long periods, set a little timer and get up at least once an hour, and preferably every 20-30 minutes. Take a break. Go get a drink of water. Go to the bathroom. Or just go say hello to the person down the hall.

Here are more easy ways to add more movement into your day:

- Park farther away from the building, whether it is your work, the grocery store or the gym.
- Carry your groceries to the car
- Take the kids to the park and *play with* them
- Take the stairs
- Carry out the trash
- Walk to the mailbox
- Take your dog for a walk

- If you are watching television, get up and move during the ads
- At the office: Stand up/Sit down several times, bend over and reach for your toes (either standing or sitting), stand up and roll your shoulders forward and back, circle your elbows, reach for the ceiling taking deep breaths. Can you think of more?

PRACTICE

What is your typical day like? Where could you reasonably add activity into your day? Write your thoughts in the space below.

MORE GOOD NEWS!

Often when we hear about how much "movement" we should be doing in a week the numbers can sound daunting. The Centers for Disease Control (CDC) recommends that American adults get at least 150 minutes of moderate aerobic activity (such as brisk walking) per week plus strength training for all major muscle groups two days per week. These exercise sessions should take place throughout the week rather than only on a few days. In other words, trying to do 75 minutes on the two weekend days is not the general idea. Instead, 30 minutes of walking five days per week is preferable. Ha! So what's the GOOD news you ask? As it turns out you can break up your 30 minutes per day into three 10-minute increments! Ten minutes seems palatable right? It doesn't have to be hard, sweaty, punishing or even time consuming. It is only 10 minutes, 3 times a day.

Here are some ways to get your 10 minutes in:

- Walk your kids to the bus stop (or to school)
- Walk around your building during a coffee or lunch break
- Walk the dog
- Take a walk with your family or friends
- Stand up out of your chair 10 times

> **Bright Idea!**
> Did you know that simply keeping track of how much you are moving can motivate you to move more? Research has shown that people who use self-monitoring tools and techniques tend to be more successful in achieving their goals. Even Benjamin Franklin set up a system of detailed grids to manage the goals he set in his plan for thirteen virtues. So, whether they are diet and exercise goals or business goals, monitoring your progress leads to success. Easy ways to monitor are keeping a journal of your activity or using a pedometer or fitness tracker.

"The word aerobics comes from two Greek words: aero, meaning 'ability to,' and bics, meaning 'withstand tremendous boredom.'"

~ DAVE BARRY

BRINGING MINDFUL AWARENESS TO MOVEMENT

There is an endless amount of information, misinformation and chatter about fitness. There is always something new and improved being introduced that is sure to be the answer to your fitness or weight loss goals.

I have been in this business long enough to see trends come and go – and then come back again! Each one promises to be the latest breakthrough in how to achieve the best results. Yes, of course there is substantial science in the world of exercise that really can optimize your results, especially if you are training for a particular event but, for our purposes, we are training for health and happiness – for life. What that means is that we must choose our movement mindfully. We want to select the types of movement that bring us joy, have limited risk of injury and allow us to continue to move throughout our lives. We must remember our individuality and respect our bodies and our specific needs. We also have to recognize that our needs will change from day to day and certainly from year to year.

I am often asked, "What is the BEST exercise?" The answer is the best-kept secret in the industry and I am about to give it to you. Get ready. This could be life changing.

The **BEST** form of exercise or movement you can do.......

Is the one you **WILL** do.

Seriously. It is that simple.

Start with what you **LIKE** to do. If you don't like it – you probably will not continue it for very long. Remember, we are in it for the long run – our lifetime.

Then, figure out what you can do. Maybe you have to begin with what you **CAN** do, to eventually enable you to do the things you like to do. That can be an amazing goal and motivator in and of itself. In other words, what types of activities do you enjoy (or at least find palatable) that you *can* do that will prepare you for those activities you really love?

What are you willing to do on a regular basis (meaning daily or several times per week)?

HERE ARE SOME EXAMPLES:

Do you like to be in nature? Maybe you would like to paint landscapes. That would mean carrying your supplies hither and yon to find a landscape to your liking. What do you need to do to get prepared to do that? Be able to walk or hike a reasonable distance? Have the strength to carry your supplies? This tells you that walking and some strength training will help you get to do the things you like with more frequency and vigor.

Maybe you would like to have more play time with your children or grandchildren. The benefits here are multifold; healthy interaction with the kids, doing something that is fun and has health benefits as well as being a role model. Of course, these activities would vary based on the age of the child/children. But here are some examples: walking or biking to a park (maybe pushing a stroller), pushing a merry-go-round, pushing (or riding) swings, going down a slide. How about some of the old fashioned games like hopscotch or jump rope? This would mean being able to walk or ride a bike a few blocks, probably carrying supplies such as water or snacks. It would mean being able to bend, climb, squat and push; perhaps a little hopping and balancing. It doesn't sound like a typical training regimen, but this is moving with the goal of doing things you love. Also, all of these things can be done without expensive equipment or going far from home.

Perhaps you want to travel to distant lands, see the world and experience different cultures. This means bags to carry and airports to walk through. There will likely be some stuffing of things in the overhead bin or under your seat, climbing onto a rental agency bus or hauling your bags along wherever you go. Travel is fun, exciting and educational. Being prepared helps you to have as much enjoyment as possible. This involves being able to walk a good distance, lift a bit of weight, bend and push, stretch and reach. What is your travel fantasy? Putting together a movement plan with your dream vacation in mind will help you make it the best trip ever!

Newly remarried in my 50s, I was enthusiastic about spending time with my new husband who loves to do all kinds of outdoor activities, particularly snow skiing. I had not skied for over 30 years, but I was willing to give it a try. I did not prepare for the demands of skiing and went out to the slopes with hope and enthusiasm. I came down from the slopes on a ski patrol medical sled with my knee blown out. (Talk about the "agony of defeat"!) After the reconstructive surgery, and having to train to learn to walk again, my patient husband and I decided that maybe cycling would be beneficial to continue my knee rehab and help keep my knee healthy long-term. I had never been a cyclist either, nor had I cared much for riding stationary cycles in the gym. The turning point came when we made a plan to go on a cycling vacation. Now that was something that sounded appealing! Vacation, quality time with my husband, combined with movement and fresh air. As I mentioned, I was NOT a cyclist. First step, get used to the idea that I would have to start getting in shape on an indoor cycle. Check. Get the right gear to make it as comfortable as possible. Check. Start slow. Double check. When the time came to think about cycling outdoors, I was really out of my element. I took several falls (13! I counted.) until I finally realized I needed professional help. After all, I was not interested in another knee injury. So I hired a cycling coach who taught me how to ride an outdoor bike, including safety, techniques for riding in traffic and around roads and hills; even using the clip-in shoes! I was able to get the hang of it well enough to make the trip and enjoy the vacation. But it should be noted that the whole process took almost a year to accomplish. Now we plan a cycling trip every year. It is the thing that keeps me motivated to get on the bike. Let me be clear. I am still NOT a "cyclist." But I have gained the skills and the ability to do something I enjoy; travel, spend time with my husband and get some exercise and fresh air, plus a nice sense of accomplishment at the end of the day.

PRACTICE

What is it **YOU LIKE** to do?

Take a few moments to ponder this. Use your imagination. Dig down and think about activities you might enjoy. Write your ideas down in the space below.

Come up with a plan to help you realize your dream. What would you need to do to carry out your plan? With as much detail as possible, describe your plan in the space below.

Hopefully, you were able to imagine an active pursuit that you will find fun and motivating. If you can, hire a professional to help you with your strategy. Having the expertise and support will make your process much easier and certainly more enjoyable. Take a lesson from my mistake. Make a plan, get professional help if needed, develop a strategy, and take the time you need to accomplish your goal. You CAN do it!

Along with this concept of selecting movement goals there is another important point to remember: WE CHANGE. Our bodies change, our life situations change, our moods change. You are not LOCKED into doing one thing for the rest of your life. You have as many choices as your imagination will allow. Movement should give you a sense of freedom and joy, not a sense of imprisonment or punishment.

The bottom line is that the most important thing you can do to encourage your lifelong health and wellness is to keep moving. Be like Goldilocks and choose the method that is JUST RIGHT for YOU.

It can be walking, cycling or water exercise. It can be yoga, Pilates or square dancing. It can be skiing, strength training or hula-hooping. It can be all of the above. You are in ultimate control. You get to decide what to do and to do what you like. Once you have made that decision, do it.

"I move, therefore I am."

~ HARUKI MURAKAMI

Ever wonder...Which is better, walking or running?
This is a trick question. Walking one mile and running one mile both burn about 100 calories. (The actual number can vary a bit due to body weight, mechanical efficiency etc.). Running gets a slight edge on the calorie burning measure because it increases the metabolic rate more than walking, so the total overall caloric burning effect of running one mile is slightly greater than walking.

However, bear in mind that the majority of us are not runners, don't like to run and probably should not choose running for basic foundational exercise. Walking on the other hand is something that most people can do, requires no equipment other than comfortable clothing and proper footwear and can be done almost anywhere. The better choice? For most of us – walking.

"Walking is man's best medicine."

~ HIPPOCRATES

COMPLETING YOUR "O"

The idea behind incorporating the concept of "O", or breath, in our discussion on life-time wellness is to illustrate how something so natural and basic can have significant impact on health and happiness. Breathing fully and deeply provides a multitude of health benefits and those benefits are multiplied when we strengthen our breath with "MM" (Mindful Movement)!

Unfortunately, our busy and often stress-filled lives upset the vital rhythm of our breath. Being mindfully aware of our need to breathe fully, frequently throughout the day and certainly during periods of stress or anxiety, can soothe our souls and reduce the negative consequences of stress. Moreover, by including mindful movement that encourages oxygen to permeate our heart, lungs and muscles we awaken the vitality that we were born with but, like water, stagnates without the flow of movement.

Getting more "O" into your day will likely require some effort, but it doesn't have to be hard. It will need to be incorporated into your day, but it doesn't have to take a significant amount of your time. It will probably take some thoughtful planning. It should not be haphazard. It will change your life and it will be worth it. It's all about the "O". Go for it!

"Remember to breathe. It is after all, the secret of life."

~ GREGORY MAGUIRE

5

W (DOUBLE-good-for-YOU) is for water

Water is the driving force of all nature.

~ LEONARDO DA VINCI

As we talked about during our first look at OWN, water makes up as much as 70% of our bodies. Here is an interesting fact; the earth is also about 70% water. Perhaps this is nature revealing to us how interconnected we are. It is easy to see that the oceans could not flourish if they were filled with coffee, diet soda, fruit juices or sports drinks. Ocean life needs water. Land animals need water. YOU need water.

We touched on some of the highlights of the benefits of water but now let's dive a little deeper (pun intended).

Hundreds of millions of years ago, when we emerged from the sea to become land dwellers, we didn't abandon the sea in favor of a different climate. No, we were born of the sea and it was part of us, intrinsically. We literally brought it with us.

Every cell in the body is filled with salt water. Plasma, the part of the blood that carries the blood cells, nutrients and waste is also salty water. Fantastically, the microscopic organisms known as mitochondria, which are inside each of our billions of cells and which allow us to utilize oxygen to make energy, were probably at one time bacteria living on their own in the vast waters that covered the earth. We brought the mitochondria with us when we became land dwellers, and they now live in the smaller, microscopic oceans of each of our billions of individual cells.

What does all this have to do with why we need water?

The point is to provide a context that allows us to somehow grasp the vital nature of water to our existence. Of course, we know we have to have water to survive. But maybe it helps to realize that it is not just that we need water. We *are* water. Without it, we literally cease to *be*.

> *"Water is life's matter and matrix, mother and medium. There is no life without water*
>
> *~ ALBERT SZENT-GYORGYI*

When we talk about all the body functions that require water, we really cannot even list them all because every function of the human body requires water.

However, just for fun, lets list some that you may know about and feel are important and maybe some that are important that you may not know about. Here we go!

BENEFITS OF WATER A TO ZIT:

A – Asthma. Water (staying hydrated) not only helps prevent asthma attacks, drinking water can help avert or diminish the severity of an asthma attack.

B – Brain. Because water is vital to all of our cellular processes, when we do not have enough water our brains suffer. Concentration, alertness, memory and the ability to do basic math are all brain functions impacted by mild dehydration.

C – Circulation (aka blood -which is a B word too). The circulation of blood delivers oxygen and nutrition to the cells and carries away waste.

D – Digestion. Drinking plenty of water helps prevent constipation and keep "things" moving.

E – Enzymes. Enzymes are catalysts for all of the chemical reactions that take place in our body and that are necessary to function. While enzymes can do their jobs without water, water helps provide a body-climate that allows enzymes to function optimally. Some examples of enzyme actions in the body include: breaking down food for digestion, DNA replication and regulating metabolism through energy production.

F – Fat & Fatigue Fighter. Drinking pure water helps increase metabolism, which burns calories and thereby fat! Water also helps fight fatigue. Fatigue, in fact, is a symptom of dehydration. Feeling sluggish? Down some H2O!

G – Gallbladder. Drink six-eight glasses of water a day to keep gallstones at bay!

H - Hair. Dehydration can affect your hair, causing brittleness and reduced shine. It has also been associated with hair loss.

I - Immune function. Dehydration suppresses your immune system. Additionally, drinking water may flush viruses from your throat to your stomach where they can't survive in the acidic stomach environment.

J – Joints. Water helps to lubricate the joints. Often people with joint pain report relief when drinking six-eight glasses of water per day.

K – Kidney. Drinking two liters of water per day can help prevent kidney stones.

L – Longevity. *F. Batmanghelidj, M.D. proclaimed, "You're not sick. You're thirsty."* In his book "Your Body's Many Cries For Water" Dr. Batmanghelidj chronicles the relationship between dehydration and many of the diseases we face that shorten our lives. Drink appropriate amounts of water to achieve maximum longevity.

M – Mood. Even mild dehydration can cause a downturn in mood, especially for women.

N – Nutrients. Water-soluble vitamins must dissolve in water in order to be absorbed. Also, plenty of water helps to excrete overdoses of these vitamins via urine.

O – Organs. Water cushions and protects vital organs.

P – Pregnancy. Water is critical to accommodate the increase in the mother's blood volume, to produce breast milk and to form the amniotic fluid that surrounds and protects the baby.

R – Respiratory system. The key word here is: MUCUS. As yucky as it sounds, your respiratory system needs water to keep its mucus moist. This not only helps in the exchange of oxygen and carbon dioxide but also in the prevention of diseases with bacterial origin (bronchitis/pneumonia) as well as reducing symptoms of COPD (chronic obstructive pulmonary disease) and cystic fibrosis.

S – Skeleton. Bones, cartilage and connective tissue all need water for strength and flexibility.

T - Temperature. Water is essential for regulating your core temperature.

U - Urinary Tract. Drinking adequate amounts of water helps keep the urinary tract free of bacteria and reduces the likelihood of a dreaded UTI (Urinary Tract Infection).

V – Vision. Some parts of our eyes are almost entirely water. Here the water helps the eye to maintain its shape, thereby impacting vision. Water is also important for tear production to lubricate the eye and rinse contaminants away.

W - Waste. The water in our bodies provides the medium to carry away waste products from our cells and tissues. In other words, it helps take out the trash. As with any trash, if not carried away these waste products can lead to disease and even death.

X - X-tras. Our muscles are about 73 percent water. They need water to contract and also to grow. Water (in the form of saliva) prevents tooth decay. Water plumps up the skin, diminishing the appearance of wrinkles.

Y – Yearning. Drinking water helps curb cravings and control hunger. Often when we get a sense of hunger or the urge to eat, we are actually thirsty. When that initial desire to eat something hits, try drinking a class of water or a cup of hot tea and see if the desire to eat is quashed for a bit.

Z – Zits. Water is good for your complexion, particularly when water takes the place of unhealthy, toxin-ridden drinks (like soda). Water helps to flush pollutants and make way for healthy skin and complexion.

"Pure water is the world's first and foremost medicine."

~ SLOVAKIAN PROVERB

I think you are getting the picture. We are basically water creatures who dwell on land. Our myriad of functions and bodily processes must use water. As a result, we have to continually provide our bodies with water for survival.

HOW MUCH WATER DO WE NEED?

The answer is: It depends. You have probably heard the general recommendation of eight 8 ounce glasses of water per day. There is actually no scientific evidence to support this. The amount of water each individual needs varies based on the size of the person, overall health status, exercise, age, environmental factors such as heat and humidity and exposure to toxins such as cigarette smoke.

Having said that, experts generally agree that eight 8 ounce glasses of water (about two liters) per day is a good guideline. Most of the people I talk to find this daunting. In our culture drinking plain water has become unappealing, boring and tasteless. This is probably because of the huge availability and billions of dollars in marketing drinks other than water, a.k.a. "anti-water." Some of the highly marketed drinks that get much more arousal response than water include: sports drinks, energy drinks, fruity drinks, soda (both diet and regular), coffee drinks, sweetened tea, beer and juices. The question everyone wants to know is, "Do these count toward my water goal for the day?"

The answer is: Not Really. While a report published by The Institute of Medicine and Academy of Sciences suggested that many people get adequate hydration from a standard diet, including caffeinated beverages, for our purposes and for optimum hydration we will not include "anti-waters" toward satisfying our water goal for the day. For the most part, beverages such as these contain loads of other ingredients that put a strain on your metabolism, contain chemicals or poisons, add unnecessary calories and contribute to inflammation in your system. Some of these added ingredients include: sugar, high fructose corn syrup, caffeine, alcohol and artificial flavors, sweeteners and colors. Overall, these kinds of "anti-water" actually cause you to need MORE water. Caffeine and alcohol are diuretics, meaning they cause you to urinate. Because you are urinating out the liquid you are ingesting, you essentially lose the opportunity to hydrate. Consequently, you need more water. Sweet beverages, even those artificially sweetened, cause inflammation, stress on the liver and increase belly fat. Overcoming the consequences of these drinks – yep you guessed it – requires more water.

Just for fun!

Pick three or four types of "anti-water" that you, your friends or your family members choose instead of water. Find the nutrition information and ingredients list on the label. Look at the ingredients. Here are some of the most common that I found*

High fructose corn syrup
Sugar
Glucose
Sucrose
Sucralose
Dextrose
Fruit Juice
Honey
Maltodextrin
Aspartame
Acesulfame potassium
Citric Acid
Phosphoric Acid
Potassium Benzoate
Caffeine
Guarana
Yellow #5
Blue #1
Red #40

*The first 11 ingredients are sweeteners.** Beware of drinks that contain added sugar OR artificial sweeteners. BOTH have been found to increase fat and inflammation.

Citric acid is a preservative. It can be used to emulsify fats and apparently is great for removing lime scale. YUM!

Phosphoric acid makes food more acidic than lemon juice and is associated with lowering bone density. It is famously known for being able to remove rust.

Potassium benzoate is a preservative that when combined with ascorbic acid degrades to a form of benzene, a known carcinogen.

Caffeine. Small amounts of caffeine have actually been shown to have some health benefits. However, the FDA has suggested that caffeine intake stay under 600mg/day. Note that your favorite coffee shop 20 oz. regular coffee contains over 400 mg of caffeine.

Guarana comes from the seeds of the guarana plant, which is known for its caffeine content. Guarana seeds contain about twice the concentration of caffeine as found in a coffee bean.

Yellow, Blue and Red are examples of added colors used to make the appearance of food more appetizing. Over the years, we have seen food dyes come and go. The reason they "Go" is because they are shown to have adverse affects including Attention Deficit Disorder (ADD) and cancer.

HOW TO GET MORE WATER INTO YOUR DAY.

I advocate getting most of your daily requirements early in the day (approximately one liter or 32 ounces). Personally, I drink 32-36 ounces before breakfast. This has a two-fold benefit; first if the goal is 64 ounces, I am more than half-way there by breakfast. It is easier to think about 10-12 ounces at lunch and dinner, and maybe eight to ten ounces worth of sips on a water bottle during the day, than trying to load up in the evening, especially before bedtime.

Also, taking this large volume of water first thing in the morning causes the stomach wall to stretch (think water balloon). This distention activates a reflex in the colon that stimulates the need to have a bowel movement. So not only are you getting much of your water needs met early in the day, you are also "clearing the way" for healthy digestion and nutrient absorption throughout the rest of day.

Unfortunately, most of us don't relish the thought of all this water. If all of those "anti-waters" don't count, what are the healthy options to meet our water needs? Here are a few suggestions along with some information as to how they can enhance your overall health and wellness as well as your water!

Lemon or Lime. Lemons and/or limes added to water may improve the flavor to your liking. Plus, you get a boost of vitamin C, which is a powerful antioxidant. It is also a widely held belief that lemons and limes help improve your body's acid/alkaline balance. This alkalinizing effect helps ward off diseases including cancer and osteoporosis.

Other fruits that may be added to water for a flavor and nutritional boost include, blueberries, raspberries and pomegranate seeds. Simply add a few berries or pomegranate seeds to a pitcher of cool water and you have a refreshing drink. Colorful berries not only taste great, they are high in antioxidants and provide support for the whole body, including eyes, brain, heart and blood sugar.

Fresh mint. Aside from its minty cool flavor, mint also has great health benefits. Long known for soothing digestive problems, mint has also been shown in animal studies to be a potential cancer fighter. It also kills bacteria, including h. pylori, salmonella and MRSA. Fresh mint can be added to cool water or used in hot water to make a soothing mint tea. Another fine feature of mint is that it grows easily. You could grow your very own mint and have all the benefits at your fingertips throughout the growing season.

Herbal Teas. Herbal teas have become a popular alternative to water or traditional tea. Each has its own flavor and benefits that are particular to the type of herb used to make the tea. Most herbal teas do not have caffeine. However, it is always best to check. Remember caffeine is a diuretic and, for our purposes, we are looking to gain hydration rather than take it away. One of my favorite herbal teas is tulsi. It is a tea brewed from Indian holy basil and documented use of tulsi has been found as early as 5000 B.C. Tulsi has been used to solve myriad health issues, including reducing symptoms of depression and promoting calm.

Decaf options. If you love your coffee or tea to the point that you must have more than 2 cups/day, consider opting for decaf on the third refill. Again, we are emphasizing a net increase in hydration. Due to the diuretic affect of caffeine, drinking regular coffee rather than water or a non-caffeinated option keeps you at zero on the hydration count.

Coconut Water. Coconut water is actually the juice of the young coconut. It has become wildly popular as both a water alternative and a sports drink. The nice thing about pure coconut water is that is tasty, additive free, caffeine free and relatively low in calories and carbohydrates. Coconut water is a natural source of potassium and magnesium, which help promote healthy blood pressure, muscles (including the heart) and bones. It should be noted that too much of these minerals can have negative side effects such as diarrhea, low blood pressure or irregular heart beat. Unless you are participating in an activity that causes you to produce a lot of sweat, keeping your coconut water intake between six to twenty ounces per day is probably sufficient.

What about other types of liquids?
Our bodies also get hydration benefits from food. Some healthful sources of food-water include soups, vegetables such as cucumbers, lettuce, cabbage, celery and carrots and watery fruits, including melons, apples and berries. It is important to keep in mind that while food-waters help provide hydration, they should be considered supplemental to your daily water routine.

"If there is magic on this planet, it is contained in water."

~ LOREN EISELEY

PRACTICE:
Think about realistic ways you can add water to your daily routine. Write down your ideas and put a plan in place. Try to get a minimum of 50 ounces of healthy, non-caffeinated fluids in each day and be true to your plan for at least seven days. Each day that you complete your plan, give yourself 10 points (and a gold star!). Give yourself an extra five points for each day that you mindfully exceed your plan by eight to ten ounces. At the end of the week: 70 points – GREAT! 100 points – OUTSTANDING!

After giving yourself a huge pat on the back, take a short self-assessment. How were your energy levels this week? Is your digestion beginning to improve? Do you see signs of your body flushing contaminants? Example: headaches, skin breakouts, muscle/joint aches. If so, don't give up! Keep up the good work until all the issues subside and you are rid of toxins. What are you willing to strive for next week?

"I believe that water is the only drink for a wise man. "

~ HENRY DAVID THOREAU

WATER WISDOM

Hopefully in our short chapter on water you are beginning to get thirsty or at least beginning to realize why water is part of OWNing your body and your power to influence your course toward a lifetime of wellness. Perhaps also you are recognizing how much water you really need to be healthy. In my household, when someone is not feeling well, one of the first questions asked is, "How much water have you had to drink?" It is a good question to ask yourself when you are feeling dull or like you might be coming down with a cold or flu.

I am very empathetic to the idea that plain water in large quantities can be hard to handle day after day after day. You are on a journey. It's time to explore options that are healthy and hydrating. The clues on your scavenger hunt for these options are to look for fluids that do not have a diuretic affect (e.g. caffeine, alcohol) and do not contain sweeteners such are those listed earlier. Wake up your taste buds with new flavors and sensations like carbonation, fruit, or even vegetables. The world is your water cooler, bring your cup, your bottle or even your own two lips and drink it up!

"In every drop of water, there is a story of life."

~ LEENA ARIF

6

N is for Nourishment

"Let food be thy medicine and medicine be thy food."

~ HIPPOCRATES

Our conversation about N centers on food (not diet), our relationship with food, and how we can develop that relationship into a healthy, enriching experience. We don't often think of food as being one of our primary relationships in life, but food is so intricately interlaced with how we experience family, friends, emotions and sense of security, that I think it is fair to say that we do "relate" with food in a variety of ways.

From an emotional standpoint, this relationship begins soon after birth in the form of how our parents choose to feed us. Ideally, feeding time is one of bonding, comforting and nurturing.

As we grew and were able to feed ourselves, did we come from an "eat everything on your plate" family? A "don't waste food" family? Or a family whose motto was "just taste it?" Furthermore, we may have experienced food as consolation, reward or even punishment. Did we get a cookie or ice cream when we suffered a loss or a disappointment? Did we get dessert for finishing our vegetables or getting good grades? How many of us were forced to sit at the table until we ate the dreaded _____(fill in the blank). If you were as stubborn as I was, you may have fallen asleep at the table when the rest of the family was already in bed!

What about family interactions? Was mealtime a time of sharing and communication, fostering family bonding, or was it stressful and angry? Did family mealtime even exist? Perhaps, like many families, the grown-ups in your family were working outside the home. This may have meant weekday meals were some form of grab-on-the-run fare in order to meet everyone's schedule.

"As a child my family's menu consisted of two choices: take it or leave it."

~ BUDDY HACKETT

Interactions with friends and food often revolve around celebration or events such as ball games, birthdays, graduations, weddings, holidays or just hanging out. Often these gatherings are centered upon food, lots of it, and often not the healthiest of choices. In many cases, such as Super Bowl parties, the entire day is highlighted by massive amounts of decadent, high calorie/low nutritive…junk. Looking at these various scenarios, we can see how our relationship with food can represent love, acceptance, support, comfort, security, celebration and friendship.

Sometimes our relationship with food can be distorted, much like an abusive relationship. We may have received messages from family, friends (or society) that food makes us fat and that fat is bad. Many of us translate those messages to mean "I am bad."

You are NOT bad, neither am I, nor is anyone else. Who we are and how we show up in our relationship with food is one of the hardest behaviors to understand and grapple with. Our feelings and actions around food play into one another. How we behave with food, e.g. overeating, binging, making bad choices, starving, purging or even over-exercising, demonstrates our level of self respect and affects our self esteem. Whether you find yourself over-filling on a celebratory meal or scarfing down a whole bag of potato chips, understanding why you are in this relationship with food is the first step in changing it, changing you – feeling better.

Some say the ability to overcome our negative behaviors associated with food is about control or discipline. While that may be true to some degree, I believe that we (our deepest essential selves) really are in a relationship with food. Think about the qualities of healthy relationships. First, we must love and respect ourselves. When we do that, we can choose to be in a relationship that is nurturing and supportive of our needs. We embrace each occasion to express love and appreciation.

If you have never thought about food in the context of a relationship, it may sound a little kooky, but stay with me on this. Healthful food, like oxygen and water, is essential for a well-functioning living being. Natural whole foods are not just healthful; they are heal-ing. When we become more mindful about the types of food we bring into our environ-ment and experiences - our homes, our families and our bodies - we make better choices and our entire being responds. Just as in any healthy relationship, our cells vibrate at a higher frequency and we exude more vitality. Our minds are brighter. Brain fog and anxi-ety disappear. It is as though a cloud has lifted and our inner being is illuminated. When we choose to care for ourselves in this way, we are demonstrating self respect. We are respecting our bodies, appreciating the quality of the substances we ingest and certainly not abusing ourselves with poisons or harmful contaminants. You see? How we interact with food is very much like other relationships. Your relationship with food is one of the most fundamental ways you can demonstrate love, specifically self-love.

> *Love yourself first and everything else falls into line. You really have to love yourself to get anything done in this world.*
>
> *~ LUCILLE BALL*

Just as with any relationship we have to know what qualities are good for us. To do that we must be curious, explore options, learn what we can and cultivate positive experi-ences with food. We must discern between what is worthy of our love and attention and what to turn our backs upon.

> *"You must learn a new way to think before you can master a new way to be."*
>
> *~ MARIANNE WILLIAMSON*

Fortunately for us, there are sincere and stalwart scientists and organizations who are dedicated to helping us make healthy and educated choices about food. What we are learning from their research is that many of the foods we grew up with are, at the very least, poor nutritional choices, and in many cases, are really quite harmful to our health. These are the food fiends we need to be wary of. Listed here are only a few examples, but the list continues to grow as we learn more and more about the importance of the type and quality of food to which we subject our ourselves and our families.

Artificial Sweeteners – These charlatans have been touted to help lose weight due to reducing calories and to be a healthy sweetener alternative for those suffering from diabetes. The fact is that artificial sweeteners have actually been shown to cause people to *gain* weight. They have also been linked to a variety of negative health problems, including migraines and metabolic syndrome - a precursor to Type 2 Diabetes.
HINT: Artificial sweeteners are NOT recommended for pregnant women. If they are bad for the unborn baby – they are probably bad for you too.

Processed Food – This is food that is commercially prepared, typically for convenience and ease of consumption. To make this food taste good, extend the shelf life and add convenience, it is generally loaded with ingredients that have been shown to be unhealthy and/or is processed to the point that it has virtually lost most of its nutritional value. Examples of processed food include: breakfast cereals, most bread, frozen dinners, frozen waffles, breakfast rolls, processed cheese products, pretzels, chips, lunch meat, salami, chicken nuggets and fruit-flavored drinks. When you think of food that is prepared, easy, convenient and fast, it is probably processed.

GMO crops/food – GMO stands for genetically modified organisms. GMO crops have been found to be toxic, allergenic and less nutritious than organically grown food. They have created problems for farmers and for the environment. Many researchers believe GMOs are associated with an uprise in a variety of illnesses that were less prevalent before the introduction of GMOs. The producers of GMO seeds claim that GMO crops are safe for consumption, however there is significant scientific evidence to the contrary. It is also worth noting that GMOs are actually banned in many countries. How do you know if it's GMO? Unfortunately, in most cases you don't. However, you can look for the Non GMO Project logo on a variety of labels to be assured (and reassured) that your selection is not genetically modified. Non GMO Project is a nonprofit organization dedicated to providing consumers with education and choices regarding GMOs.

"Bad Fats" – Fats on the "Bad" list include canola oil, corn oil, vegetable shortening, hydrogenated oil, partially hydrogenated oil, soy bean oil and trans-fats. Individually, each of these fats has characteristics that can actually cause disease. Generally, these fats increase inflammation in your body, which is associated with every disease, particularly heart disease, stroke, cancer, diabetes and autoimmune diseases.

Sugar – We think of sugar as that white stuff that we add when we bake cookies and cakes to make them sweet. However, sugar comes in many forms and is found in our foods in alarming amounts. Some other names for sugar are: "natural sugar", high fructose corn syrup, fructose, agave, honey, dextrose, sucralose and fruit juice. While some of these sugars are worse than others (particularly fructose and high fructose corn syrup), none of them are "sweet nothings." Here is a list of some of the romances they are whispering in your ear:

> "Psssst. We cause heart damage, belly fat, obesity, cancer, diabetes, liver dam-age and dementia. We **know** you love us. You can never give us up! You are **addicted** to us..."

That's right. That is the scary part about sugar. It IS addictive and the food industry knows this. That is why we find sugar in almost every processed food. It is in your hot dog, the ketchup, the relish and the bun! Something you thought was not sweet at all actually contains a fair amount of sugar. When you consider how many "non-sweet" foods contain sweeteners, if you are eating processed food it really adds up.

What is even more diabolical about our sweet friend is that it is linked to so many devastating illnesses. While we have often associated sugar with obesity and diabetes, it might surprise you to know that sugar is the primary food source for cancer cells.

If you are interested in learning more about healthy food and a healthy planet, check out some of these resources:
Robert Wood Johnson Foundation http://www.rwjf.org/en.html
Healthy Eating Research http://healthyeatingresearch.org
Physician's Committee for Responsible Medicine http://www.pcrm.org
Environmental Working Group http://www.ewg.org
Institute for Responsible Technology http://responsibletechnology.org
Earth Open Source http://earthopensource.org
Center for Science In The Public Interest http://cspinet.org/about/index.html
GreenMedInfo Education Equals Empowerment http://www.greenmed info.com

Gluten and friends. – In recent years there has been a lot of discussion and even some controversy about problems with gluten in foods. What is gluten? It is a protein that is made up of two small proteins called gliadin and glutenin. It is found naturally in wheat, barley, rye and a newcomer to this list, triticale. Of course, we can find gluten in products like cereals and breads made from these grains, but it has become a pervasive food additive due to its ability to add elasticity to dough, enhance the texture of foods and as a stabilizing additive in processed foods such as ice cream and ketchup. While there is still a camp of dietitians and physicians that believes gluten-containing foods are acceptable, more and more health professionals are recommending against it. Many gastroenterologists globally are recommending that gluten actually be eliminated from the diet. While it is difficult to pinpoint all of the damage that gluten causes, it has been strongly associated with digestive disorders, cardiorespiratory problems, allergies and even psychological disorders. There are several problems associated with gluten in our food. Problem number one is that gluten, like sugar, is in SO many products. It is in everything from caramel coloring to hot cocoa to deli meats and beer. If the food is processed – it probably has gluten. Problem number two is that gluten does not only come from wheat but also from rye, barley and triticale. Therefore, as a consumer you have to be aware of multiple gluten containing grains, not just wheat. Problem number three is the argument that how the grains are grown (organic vs. conventional) makes a significant difference in whether they are a contributor to the problems associated ingesting them. However, the extensive research in this area supports the idea that gluten is the primary culprit and conventional farming simply adds insult to injury. Sadly, the food industry is onto us in a big way. We now see the supermarket shelves teeming with "gluten-free" products. This is reminiscent of the "fat-free" fad years ago. That clever food industry knows we can't give up our breads, cakes, pies and cookies, so they have created gluten-free ways for us to get our fix. While these foods may not contain gluten, they contain other forms of refined carbohydrates (rice and potato starch) and sugars. From a whole person health perspective, these products spike blood sugar, causing an insulin response that can lead to all the damaging affects of sugar, including type 2 diabetes, heart disease and cancer. Consider reducing your intake of these types of foods; maybe consider them as a special treat rather than a staple or perhaps avoid them altogether. If your daily bread is a prime source of happiness for you, there are many healthful bake at home recipes that utilize alternative no-gluten ingredients such as buckwheat, chia, oats and coconut butter to provide the loaf of comfort you desire.

TIME TO BREAK UP

Having an unhealthy relationship with the foods mentioned above is toxic and debilitating. These foods will drain your life and energy. Turn your back on them and move on. You are on the road to feel-good town and these foods will only slow you down.

Now, let's think back and remember what it feels like to have a cherished, loving relationship. You might imagine it is very much like a relationship with your own newborn baby. The newness of it can be exciting! It feels good to care for something of supreme importance, a new life. You *want* to make all the best choices so that your newborn can have the best opportunities that life can offer. One of the most vital and impactful areas where we can make a difference in this new and budding life is through our choice of food.

We know that natural, whole foods are life giving. They are nurturing from the inside out. They offer nourishment, promise health and well being, cleanse impurities, prevent disease and allow the body to flourish. Wholesome food supports growth, fosters a healthy mind and provides a foundation from which a person can develop and achieve her/his highest potential.

Isn't that what we want in a healthy relationship?

YES!

HOW DO WE FIND THIS DREAM-RELATIONSHIP?

Let's take a look at some considerations in our quest for a healthy relationship with food.

DIET IS A FOUR-LETTER WORD.

> *"Food is like sex: when you abstain, even the worst stuff begins to look good."*
>
> *~ BETH MCCOLLISTER*

Unless your physician has put you on a medically supervised diet – DON'T DIET. Try to avoid even using the word, much less actually "going on" one! Being "on a diet" is like being in jail. Once you are in it, all you want is out. All you can think about is what you can do and have once you are out of jail. What does this lead to? JAILBREAK! We "misbehave", and eat whatever it is we have been craving, and eventually we end up back in jail. Diets don't work in the long run, and for most of us, actually lead to weight gain over time.

Consider this your "Get Out of Jail Free" card. Fly away! Don't look back!

We have already talked about some of the foods to turn your back on. Now let's look at how to find healthy food and make good choices. Here are some things to consider when choosing food:

DOES IT HAVE A LABEL?

In a nutritiously perfect world, we would eat food that is not processed or with limited human-made adjustments. The label test is simply to identify how much processing the food has undergone. For example, when you buy an apple, the only thing on it is a sticker that tells you the type of apple and whether it is organic or conventional (unless of course you buy straight from the grower, which is extra "good-for you!" points). When you buy an apple cake, there is a label with a list of ingredients that went in to processing the cake. Generally speaking, the fewer the ingredients and the more "whole" the food is (in other words, less chopping, juicing, mashing etc.), the more nutritious the food. Of course there are exceptions to this. But if you are a beginning label reader/ healthy food buyer, this is a simple way to think about it. The idea is to select food with the least amount of processing and added ingredients as possible. Consider this, often the list of ingredients that you can't pronounce is there to increase the shelf life of the product. While these ingredients keep the food palatable for a longer period of time, they are typically not great for your health and in larger amounts can be toxic. So while adding these ingredients may give the product a longer shelf life, it doesn't do anything for yours.

Did you know?
Fruits and vegetables are not all that different from us. When we cut or chop them, they begin to lose some of their vital energy, not unlike how we bleed when we are cut.

Foods that are precut and packaged so that we don't have to do the chopping ourselves have already begun to seep out some of the goodness. Ideally, try to do your cutting and chopping right before your plan to eat the food.

FALL IN LOVE WITH HEALTHY FOOD.

Have you, or someone you know, ever experienced a bad relationship, fallen in love with the wrong person; eventually figured out the mistake in judgment, successfully gotten out of the relationship, only to fall in love with another big mistake? It is not uncommon that we are attracted to something in a relationship that seems sexy and exciting at the time, but eventually leads to disappointment and regret. To find the right relationship for us we need to look for qualities that are wholesome, respectful, supportive and long-lasting. This may mean we need to change our minds about what we find attractive.

The same is true for food. Oh, we are so enamored with the double chocolate fudge brownie, the bacon cheeseburger and the chili cheese fries, but these and others like them are all the same. They are treacherous and disloyal. They promise comfort and satisfaction, but in the long run they provide nothing but obsession, craving and remorse. At the time they may feel like all contentment and coziness, but in the end they are unkind, they hurt us and make us feel badly about ourselves. We have to break up with those noxious foods and look for high quality, virtuous food. This is not easy because our minds (and taste buds) have learned to like a certain thing. It means we have to recognize the virtues we desire in food and be willing to sample new and unfamiliar colors, flavors, textures – personalities.

"Every new beginning comes from some other beginning's end."

~ SENECA

Trying out new kinds of healthy food can be both scary and fun. It is similar to the cereal commercial where the little boys don't want to try the new cereal because it is supposed to be good for you. Oh! It is so hard to turn our backs on our favorite things and to try things we are certain can't taste good and, even if they do, they must be too hard to prepare, too expensive, too hard to find or other rationales for not trying them. The thing is, if you don't step out of your comfort zone and try new things, you will never grow. Remember our wellness quote, *Wellness is a conscious commitment to* **growth and improvement in all areas."** If we don't grow, we stagnate and stagnation leads to deterioration and decay. Exploring new ways to nurture your body through healthy food and eating habits can be exciting and awakening. Have courage. There will be those things that are simply not for you, but over time you will discover a whole new world of food that is beautiful, enticing, tasty AND good for you!

"And the day came when the risk to remain tight in a bud was more painful than the risk it took to blossom."

~ ANAIS NIN

I want to encourage you to move forward with an open heart and mind. Just as it is hard to give up a fouled relationship, it is a challenge to let go of those dreadfully nasty foods. As with any relationship, those offensive foods actually become a part of us. REALLY! We are attached to them. They influence our DNA. We truly ARE what we EAT. Because of this, it can take some time for us to be attracted to other foods with different personalities. A healthy-food rival may actually taste bad the first (or second or third!) time we try it. With time, patience and determination however, our taste buds and our viewpoints change. We may actually return to a food that once made our taste buds wince to find something we truly enjoy! As we persevere we are embracing our self esteem, self respect and self efficacy. We practice mindful aware-ness as we consider food that will nurture us on every level; physical, mental, emo-tional and spiritual.

People who know me now would never guess that there was a period in my life, many years ago (more like an era!), when my diet consisted of 1-2 liters of diet soda per day, candy bars, chips, ice cream sandwiches, pizza and the oh-so-coveted green chile cheeseburger. YUM! I was hooked on peanut M&Ms and never went anywhere without a handful in my pocket. If you were to meet me now, you would never imag-ine such a thing.

Don't get the wrong idea; I did not give all these things up at once, and giving them up completely actually took years. But I can tell you that I do not long for my lost relationship with them. I never think of that time as "the good old days". I do not have cravings of any sort. Indeed, I am so sensitive to the taste of sweet that some salad dressings, dried fruit and even some vinegars are utterly distasteful to me.

To reach this point in my personal journey has taken the better part of my life. It has been educational, thought provoking and illuminating. My overall health and well-being are better than they have ever been, and I am so appreciative of all the circumstances (as challenging as some of them were) that have led me to this place in my life. But wellness is not a destination; it is a journey, an on-going process that lasts a lifetime. I am continuing along my path and am pleased to be able share what I have learned with you.

> *"So long as there is breath in me, that long will I persist. For now I know one of the greatest principles of success; If I persist long enough I will win."*

> *~ OG MANDINO*

POWERFUL YOU. YOU HAVE THE POWER TO CHOOSE WELL

How do we define good food? Good food is that which is loving, supportive and nurturing to our entire being and to our planet. How do we know what that IS? It can be so confusing. We get so many messages from the food industry marketers who know we are looking for information. They prey on our psychology for their gratification from huge profits. Add to that the fact that the information we get from health news is constantly changing; one day eggs are bad, margarine is good – the next day eggs are good, margarine is bad. One day whole grains are recommended, the next day everything is gluten-free. Good fats, bad fats! Good carbs, bad carbs! Protein; too much or too little? Who can make sense of it all? **YOU CAN and I am here to help!**

Next up is some basic information that will help you in making your selection of *good foods*:

EAT YOUR COLORS – AKA "THE GOOD CARBS"

This does not pertain to things like orange soda and cheese puffs. Eating your colors refers to vegetables and fruits. Soda, chips, bread, pasta, as well as broccoli, yams and bananas, all belong to the broad category of food we call carbohydrates. "Carbs" have gotten a pretty bad reputation over the past few years, so I think it is important to realize that not ALL carbs are bad. The Good Carbs are those that are typically nature-made and possess color and fiber. A fun and easy way to remember the Good Carbs is to think of them as a natural-food-rainbow; red, orange, yellow, green, blue, indigo and violet. What foods match these colors?

Red: Beets, apples, raspberries, tomatoes, radishes, strawberries, pomegranates, red bell peppers

Orange: Oranges, papaya, yam/sweet potato, pumpkin, grapefruit, carrots

Yellow: Squash, lemons, peaches, yellow peppers, pineapples, mangos, yellow beets

Green!: Greens are super food. Darker the green – typically a better choice. Broccoli, avocado, spinach, kale, cilantro, parsley, asparagus, chard, peas, brussel spouts, bok choy

Blue/Indigo/Violet: Eggplant, blueberries, blackberries, plums, black olives, prunes, purple carrots, purple cauliflower, purple grapes, purple figs

While a general rule of thumb is that colors are better, there are some tremendously healthful foods that are pale in color. Some prime examples are: cauliflower, mushrooms (especially Japanese varieties), onion, garlic and ginger. Be sure to include these in your cooking for both flavor and nutrition.

A cautionary note on fruit

As you can see from our list of colorful Good Carbs above, fruit is among some of the most colorful and tasty! For ages we have been told how wonderfully healthy and wholesome fruits are. Indeed, most colorful fruits like those listed above have pretty powerful nutritional qualities. Because fruit requires very little preparation (if any), and is certainly delicious, we feel pretty good about eating it. However, fruit is also naturally sweet – that's why we love it so much! The primary sugar in fruit is fructose which occurs as part of nature, unlike high fructose corn syrup found in many processed foods. Research is telling us that our bodies metabolize fructose differently than glucose. Too much fructose puts a strain on the liver and is converted to fat more readily than glucose. (Glucose is the primary sugar-produced in metabolism of carbohydrate food; those foods that are not protein or fat.) Also, when we eat foods that contain fructose, the parts of the brain that make us feel full are not affected, so we don't get a message from the brain that tells us we are full. The result is, we eat too much and most of it is turned to fat. Health experts caution that we should not eat more than 25 grams of fructose per day, and even less than that for many people. How do we translate that to actual fruit? To give you some idea of how this translates into real food, eating one medium apple, one medium banana and less than a cup of blueberries translates to approximately 25 grams of fructose.

What to do? Here are some simple recommendations.

First, remember these important points.

1. Fresh is typically better.
2. Variety is wondrous. All the colors of fruit have delightful benefits so enjoy them – in moderation.
3. Avoid most fruit juices, nectars and canned fruit of any sort. We have been misled into believing that fruit juices are a healthy option. But truly, most packaged fruit juices have the "healthy" processed out of them. They lose many of their nutrients and fiber, leaving you with a fructose-sweet fruit drink that your body doesn't metabolize well.
4. *Be mindful* and *pay attention* to the amount of fruit you are eating. When in doubt, check it out. If you are interested, you can find complete lists of foods and their fructose levels with an easy Internet search.

Speaking of Juice – the OJ Story Revealed

For almost half a century, orange juice has been a staple as a healthy breakfast juice choice and a vitamin C-packed-sunshine-in-a-glass super food. As it turns out, we have been duped. The orange juice that we see on the shelves at the grocery store is far from healthful and, in fact, can contribute to many illnesses including metabolic syndrome, diabetes and arthritis.

Here is the down and dirty on OJ. First, as with any fruit, oranges have a growing season. They do not grow all year long on magical trees in Florida. As a result, in order to keep OJ on the shelf year-round something has to be done to preserve it. The process involves removing the juice from the oranges, storing the juice in huge tanks, many of which can hold over a million gallons. Once in the tanks, a process takes place the removes oxygen from the juice. The "deoxygenation" allows the juice to be stored for over a year without spoiling. Unfortunately, this process also removes the yummy orange taste that we think of when with think of OJ.

(sigh) What's a manufacturer to do? Stuck with millions of gallons of juice that is tasteless and colorless (that's right – no orange-orange juice), manufacturers must turn to experts in the fields of color, smell and flavor in order to concoct your favorite orangey breakfast beverage. Who are these people? They are chemists who are experts in how to get the pleasure centers in your brain to light up with just the right sweetness, citrusy-orange scent and sunshiny hue to make you feel like you are really drinking fresh squeezed sunshine-in-a-glass orange juice. To add insult to injury, the chemicals used in creating this potion are often imported from other countries that may be using toxic chemicals or pesticides in their products. Food manufacturers are not required to divulge these additives on their labels. As a consumer, you have no idea what you are actually drinking.

But wait! It gets worse!

Just when you thought the news couldn't get much worse, it actually does. When we consider the tasty sweetness of most juices, we must realize that our bodies translate the sweetness in the juice just as though it is table sugar. But it is worse than table sugar, because juice is primarily fructose. An 8 oz. glass of orange juice has almost the some amount of sugar as a can of soda.

This creates a tremendous load on the liver and pancreas. The science tells us that, ultimately, drinking sweet juices causes us to eat more calories, increase belly fat and increase risk of Type 2 Diabetes and heart disease.

What to do?

All of this does not mean we can't support our friends in the orange growing industry. We can select and eat delicious organic whole oranges when they are in season and get the benefits of the whole fruit, including: fiber, vitamins C, B1, B9 (folate), A and a healthy blend of minerals as well.

For more detailed information, check out "Squeezed: What You Don't Know About Orange Juice", by Alissa Hamilton.

Glycemic Index. What is it ? Why should you care?

According to the University of Sydney, glycemic index (GI) is a way of ranking food on a scale from 1 to 100 based on the degree to which they cause blood sugar levels to rise after eating. Foods with a high GI are digested and absorbed rapidly, which causes blood sugar levels to dramatically spike and drop (imaging a crazy roller coaster ride!) Conversely, low-GI foods are digested and absorbed more slowly and produce gradual rises in blood sugar and insulin levels. Low GI foods are a necessary part of a healthful diet. According to the On Line Glycemic Index Database (http://www. Gilisting.com), low GI foods are 55 GI or below, Medium GI foods are 56-69 and High GI foods are 70 and above.

A newer term that may be helpful to know and understand is Glycemic Load (GL). Glycemic load is a way to categorize foods in a way that takes into consideration both the amount of carbohydrate in a certain food and its effect on blood sugar (GI).

GL is determined by multiplying the GI by the number of grams of carbohydrates/100. Don't worry; unless this is a recipe you have made at home, you don't have to do the math. If you are interested in the GL of a certain food, it can be found easily on the Internet. However, for the sake of illustration, let's take a look at a few common foods. You can imagine that the GI & GL of certain foods such as cakes, cookies, sodas, candy and white breads are going to be high. Just for fun, let's play a game. Look at some common foods and guess which has a higher GI/GL. Below is a list of pairs of foods. Circle the one you think has the *lower* GI/GL of the two:

1.	Corn on the Cob	Grapes
2.	Baked Russet Potato	Sweet Potato
3.	Brown Rice	White Rice
4.	Fruit Roll Up	M&Ms Peanut
5.	Apple Juice	Orange Juice
6.	Corn Tortilla	Flour Tortilla
7.	Rice Cakes	Rye Crips
8.	Fettuccini	Lender's Bagel
9.	Banana	Pear
10.	Shredded Wheat	Kellogg's Corn Flakes

Answers: 1. Grapes 2. Sweet potato 3. Brown rice 4. M&Ms 5. Apple juice 6. Corn tortilla 7. Rye crisps
8. Fettuccini 9. Pear 10. Shredded wheat

Interesting observation – According to the International Table of Glycemic Index and Load, many international companies seemingly sell the same products such as cereals, crackers and breads in multiple countries. In researching glycemic index however, I found the GI of foods sold in the United States higher than the same foods sold under the same label in other countries. It would appear that food manufacturers add more sugar to foods sold in the U.S. than foods sold in other countries.

Choosing the best fruits can be a little complicated when you are trying to take into consideration both the fructose level and the glycemic index. Try not to get too bolloxed up in absolute do's and don'ts. Simply limit your fruit consumption remembering your best choices are those with the highest nutrient value that are also lower in fructose and glycemic index. I hear you. Now we are back to being overwhelmed and confused. Not to worry, here are some examples:

Best: Avocados, Kiwi, Grapefruit, Strawberries, Raspberries
Good: Apricots, Plums, Peaches, Blueberries,
Fair: Apples, Pears, Oranges, Red Grapes,
Limited amounts only: Bananas, Figs, Dried Fruit, Watermelon

When it comes to carbohydrates, remember the good guys. It is important to keep in mind that there are thousands of really super-healthy foods that fall under the category of "Carbohydrate." Remember this when you hear people talking about "Low-carb" diets. The nourishing carbohydrates in the vegetables and fruits we have been discussing are essential for our bodies to keep us humming along in optimum health.

NEXT UP. PROTEIN.

We have heard a lot of confusing information about protein over the years. Dietitians told us we had too much protein in our diets and needed to cut back, and then came all the varieties of high protein diets; we were warned about those as well (and probably rightfully so). How should we go about getting the right amount of protein with our daily food choices and what kinds of protein are best?

First, it helps to know why protein is important. Protein is foundational to practically every function of the human body. It plays an elemental role in immune function, muscles and movement, hormones and structural support; from cell membranes to bones. Proteins are also necessary for transporting nutrients to the cells and also every chemical reaction in the body. Bottom line: Our bodies need protein. Additionally, our protein needs will fluctuate throughout our lifetimes. Certain times in our lives we need more protein than others, such as:

- Periods of growth – including childhood and pregnancy
- Periods of stress

- Recovery from injury
- As we age (Women and men over 45 need more protein to prevent muscle wasting)
- Periods of increased physical activity

Where do we get protein in our diet and what types of protein are good choices? Good sources of protein can come from both animal and plant sources. The idea of a good source of protein has to do with the number of essential amino acids in the protein. Amino acids are the building blocks of protein. There are twenty amino acids and nine of them are considered "essential." During certain periods of growth or illness a tenth amino acid, arginine, is also considered to be essential. They are called essential because the body cannot manufacture them; we have to include them in the food we eat. Animal sources of protein such as eggs, meat, poultry and seafood contain all essential amino acids and are considered "complete" proteins. Plants can also be terrific sources of quality protein. However, most fruits and vegetables do not contain complete protein, which has led to the concept of vegetarians having to include various combinations of foods each day in order to get all the essential amino acids. In recent years, as more and more Americans have been choosing a vegetarian diet we have discovered that some plant sources do have complete protein. These include quinoa, buckwheat, amaranth, soy, chia, hempseed, blue-green algae and spirulina.

MAKING SENSE OUT OF HOW MUCH PROTEIN YOU NEED

As mentioned earlier, our protein needs vary, not just during different periods of our life but also from day to day. This is especially true if you are a regular exerciser. To get a feel for how much protein you need, let's go through some simple calculations. Please know that this information is generalized for the purposes of this book to simply give you an idea of how much protein you may need in your food plan.

To begin, we need to calculate your body weight in kilograms (kg). Don't worry, a simple calculator will do.

1. Calculate your body weight in kilograms (kg)

Body Weight lbs._____ / 2.2 = _____ Body Weight kg

2. Determine your activity level

Below you will find a table that provides suggested protein requirements per day. Along the left hand column find your age. Across the top of the table find your activity level.

1= sedentary, an occasional walk or light activity

2= moderately active, walking (or similar exertion level) 3-5 times/week

3=very active, strenuous exercise more than 3times/week + moderate activity most days of the week

4=athlete in training

3. Determine your age group

Find your age group on the left and your activity level across the top. Now, run your finger across horizontally from your age and down vertically from your activity level. The number you see there is an estimate of the amount of protein in grams you need for each kg that you weigh.

4. Calculate your estimated daily protein requirements

Take that number _____g X Body Weight kg _____ = Estimated amount of protein in grams (g) that you need each day.

Example:

Kim is a moderately active 45 year old who weighs 140lbs:

140lbs/2.2= 63.64kg

Multiply 1.2g/kg X 63.64 = roughly 74g of protein needed per day *

Remember to be like Goldilocks and choose the number that most represents YOUR needs.

RECOMMENDED DAILY PROTEIN INTAKE

(Grams of Protein Per Kilogram Body Weight)

AGE	ACTIVITY LEVEL			
	1	2	3	4
20 - 44	.8 – 1.0	1.0 – 1.1	1.2 – 1.3	1.4 – 1.7+
45 – 64	.9 – 1.1	1.1 – 1.3	1.3 – 1.4	1.5 – 1.7+
65 and over	1.0 – 1.2	1.2 – 1.4	1.4 – 1.5	1.5 – 1.7+

Now back to our regularly scheduled program of making sense of it all.

OK. We figured out our approximate daily protein needs. What does that mean in terms of our daily food intake?

Here are some examples of quality protein sources:

Food	Qty.	Protein Grams
Eggs	1 large	6
Beef	3 oz.	22
Chicken Breast	½	30
Fish (Salmon)	3 oz.	19
Beans (Pinto)	1 cup	15
Nuts (Almonds)	20 nuts	4
Whey	1 oz.	20
Soybeans	1 cup	29
Organic Tofu	½ cup	10
Organic Tempeh	½ cup	15
Quinoa (Cooked)	1 cup	8
Buckwheat (Cooked)	1 cup	5.5
Amaranth (Cooked)	1 cup	9
Chia	1 oz.	4
Spirulina	2 Tbsp.	8
Greek Yogurt	6 oz.	17

Note: A 3 oz. serving of meat is about the size of a deck of cards.

In our example, Kim needs 74g of protein per day. You can see by looking at the protein sources in the table that getting enough good quality protein can require some forethought and mindful decision-making. Let's look at some options for Kim:

Breakfast:	(1) 6 oz. carton of plain Greek yogurt and fresh fruit	= 17g
Snack:	10 Almonds	= 2g
Lunch:	Salad with ½ chicken breast	= 30g
Dinner:	4 oz. Salmon filet	= 25g
Total Protein for the Day		74g

Key points to remember on protein needs:
Research on protein requirements is varied and does not provide a hard and fast rule. However, the key points listed below give you a solid framework for meeting your daily protein requirement. If you are dealing with a special situation, such as an illness or specific sports training regimen, I recommend you meet with a registered dietitian to get a precise assessment of your personal needs.

1. .80 grams of protein per kilogram body weight is the MINIMUM requirement. Many health professionals believe our needs are greater that that.
2. MORE is NOT necessarily BETTER. Taking in excessive amounts of protein well beyond your daily needs simply adds calories to the day and will likely be stored as fat and can put stress on your kidneys.
3. It is BEST to spread your protein intake throughout the day. Your body can only absorb so much protein at a time. A general rule of thumb is about 30g of protein per meal/snack. This number can vary depending on the type of protein and the intensity of a person's exercise routine. By taking in too much at one sitting you are wasting calories and money.
4. You can see from the table that as we age we actually need more protein in order to preserve our muscle mass and stay healthy.
5. Too much protein can be harmful to your kidneys. If you have a history of kidney problems and are taking in large quantities of protein, you should see a medical professional to ensure your kidneys are functioning properly.
6. These general guidelines do not take gender into account. The reason for this is that to truly get an accurate picture (for those who feel they need

it), we need to know the percentage of our body weight that is not coming from fat. Men typically have more muscle mass than women. In this scenario, we account for that difference by using body weight in our calculations. If this information has you really jazzed about getting the right amount of protein in your diet, find a registered dietitian or a nationally certified personal trainer in your area. Barring any medical considerations you may have, either should be able to calculate your fat free mass and give you a more precise measure of your protein needs.

PRACTICE

Use the calculations and tables above to estimate your daily protein needs. Next, write down what you ate yesterday. Did you get enough protein? Too much?

Now create 2-3 days of menus (like we did for Kim) that would give you adequate protein (with the appropriate amount in each meal ~ 30 g) variety and taste good!

FAT
One-Fat, Two-Fat, Red-Fat, Blue-Fat

Fat is where it's at!

Fat is the third of the big three in our nourishment discussion on choosing the best foods. Poor fat. It has been maligned and misunderstood for decades. Popular diets have centered on the idea that fat going in your body will wind up as fat showing up on your belly, hips and thighs.

I remember the low-fat era. I completely bought into the idea that fat was the devil. The concept, which seemed reasonable at the time, was that ounce per ounce, fat had more calories than its leaner companions, carbohydrates and protein. From a simply caloric standpoint this made a lot of sense. However, research surfaces almost daily that proves this concept to be wrong. The fact is that our bodies NEED fat. Our brains and nervous systems are primarily fat. Fat cushions and protects our organs. Our bodies need fat to absorb vitamins A, D, E, and K and much more.

> *"No diet will remove all the fat from your body because the brain is entirely fat. Without a brain you might look good, but all you could do is run for public office."*
>
> *~ GEORGE BERNARD SHAW*

If you have been depriving yourself of fat because you were told it was bad for you, REJOICE! Fat is not only good for you, it is necessary! There is one caveat. We need to choose GOOD fat. Yes, there are different types of fat. Some are very very good and some are horrid. To enjoy all the flavor and benefits of fat, again we must make informed choices about the foods we eat and how we prepare them.

LET'S LOOK AT THE YUCKY STUFF FIRST.
Hydrogenated/Partially Hydrogenated Fat/Trans-fat* – These types of fat are created by forcing hydrogen into animal or vegetable fat. They have been widely used because they are cheap and they increase the shelf life of food. Hydrogenated oils are a type of fat that can withstand very high temperatures and are often used for frying. These characteristics are the reason vegetable shortening, margarine, prepackaged foods, fast foods, doughnuts, non-dairy toppings and creamers tend to be loaded with

hydrogenated oils. Any oil can be hydrogenated, and even ordinary vegetable oils will convert to trans-fat during frying. Some of the more commonly hydrogenated oils are corn, peanut, soybean and cottonseed.

*The FDA has determined that trans-fats are not considered safe in any amount. Effective June 2018, trans-fats may no longer be added to or used in food processing. **Bottom line** – Avoid these oils and products that contain them.

Canola Oil – Canola oil deserves a dishonorable mention all its own. Canola oil is genetically engineered rapeseed oil. Rapeseed is inexpensive to grow because it is toxic to insects and therefore doesn't require costly pesticides. The toxic ingredient in rapeseed oil is Erucic Acid. The genetic engineering of the rapeseed oil decreases the percent of erucic acid in the oil to make it more palatable for human consumption. Rapeseed has so many negative characteristics that manufacturers need to add hexane to extract oil from the seed, along with various chemicals used for bleaching, refining and degumming and deodorizers used to hide its foul-smell when exposed to high heat. **Bottom line** – If you have it in your cupboard, throw it away. Avoid products containing any form of canola oil.

GOOD FAT TO THE RESCUE!

There are so many delicious and good for you oils, you need never feel deprived again. Here is a list of several wonderful options. Alongside each is just a bit of information to help you incorporate them in the most beneficial way.

Coconut Oil – Coconut oil is currently thought of as one of the best fats you can have in your diet. Why? It is anti-microbial and anti-viral. It is not only recommended for use in cooking but can also be added to smoothies, coffee, toast or used in any other way your palate desires. But wait! Coconut oil can also be used topically as a moisturizer, conditioner, mouth rinse, deodorant and more! The properties of coconut oil make it healthy for your brain and gut. It can withstand high heat cooking and does not go rancid. **Bottom line** - Coconut oil gets 5 stars. Add it to your daily food routine. Look for organic virgin or extra virgin.

Olive Oils – Most of us are familiar with the benefits of olive oil from all the publicity surrounding the Mediterranean Diet and heart health. While there has been some confusion about high temperature cooking with olive oil, the International Olive Council has stated that olive oil can withstand high temperature without denaturing to an unhealthy state. Nevertheless, I suggest keeping your sautéing at medium temperatures, just to be on the safe side. **Bottom Line** - Use olive oil abundantly for many of your cooking needs. You may prefer higher quality, robust olive oil for salad dressings and dipping and the lighter olive oil for light sautéing and frying.

Avocado – Avocado oil has very similar properties to olive oil, which makes it a healthy choice for dressings and for cooking. The avocado itself has a number of health benefits besides its oil; avocados are abundant in fiber, minerals, anti-oxidants and vitamins. **Bottom Line** – Yes, avocado oil is great – but the whole avocado is loaded with good stuff like fiber, vitamins and minerals, so enjoy the whole thing regularly!

Nuts & Seeds – To understand the beauty of nuts and seeds, it helps to remember that nuts and seeds contain the DNA of the plant. Specifically, seeds contain the essence of the life of the plant. As with avocado, nuts and seeds have tremendous health benefits. Recent research looking at the benefits of eating nuts has shown that nuts of all sorts are beneficial in reducing cancer risk to treating erectile dysfunction and everything in between. The nuts and seeds we see most commonly are: almonds, pecans, walnuts, cashews, pistachios, sesame seeds, flax seeds and chia. Using nut oils in preparing deliciously healthy meals can be a tasty treat. But remember that nut oils can be expensive and do not maintain their goodness in high heat, with the exception of sesame oil. **Bottom Line** - Eat a wide variety of nuts and seeds to get the benefit of the whole food. When cooking using seed oil, choose sesame oil.

Fish oil – The primary compounds in fish oil that make it crucial to our health are the omega 3 fatty acids. Fish oil and omega 3 fatty acids have been associated with improved heart health, brain health, reduced inflammation, improvement in childhood behavioral disorders, eye health, arthritis and more! Most physicians agree that we should have an ample amount of high quality fish oil/omega 3 fatty acids in our daily food plan. Examples of good sources of fish oil include: wild salmon, pacific mackerel, cod, blue fin tuna and rainbow trout. The key is to select fish with the lowest possibility of contaminants such as mercury and industrial pollutants. A general rule of thumb is that the larger the fish the more highly contaminated. Fish oil can also be taken in supplement form. The fish oil from supplements can also be contaminated, so be sure to look for a high quality fish oil and do your research to make sure the source of the fish oil is as clean as possible. **Bottom line** - Our bodies must have omega 3 fatty acids and fish oil is a prime source. Try to include fish oil in your daily routine.

Flax Seeds and Flaxseed Oil – Along with chia, flax is prized by many vegetarians as one of the best plant-based sources of omega 3 oil. Unfortunately, the type of fat in flax is not readily usable as omega 3 in the body. Therefore, the body has to use the building block fat in flaxseed to manufacture the preferred omegas (like those found in fish). This is not a very efficient process, which leaves vegetarians really needing to be mindful about how to get their recommended amount of omega 3s. The other element that flax is famous for is called lignan. Lignans are known for their high fiber content, antioxidant qualities and ability to regulate hormones. Flaxseed oil should not be used for cooking because the heat damages the beneficial properties of the oil. From a nutritional standpoint, the flaxseeds win out over flax oil due to their fiber, protein, mineral and vitamin content. Be aware that our digestive system doesn't break down the flax seed very well. Consequently, it has more nutrient availability if is it ground before eating. You can buy ground flax seed or toss a bit in a coffee grinder and grind it up right before you use it. **Bottom line** - Do try to include some flax as part of your healthy fat intake. To get the most out of your flax, be mindful of the precautions noted above.

Chia Seeds – Chia seeds pack such a powerful punch they deserve a heading all their own. Chia is a quality source of protein, fiber, vitamins and minerals and, like flaxseed, can be a source of omega 3 fat as well. The ancient Mayans relied on chia for strength and endurance. All of these great benefits come at a very low caloric cost. **Bottom Line** - Chia is a great addition to a variety of recipes including breads, smoothies, pizza crust, salads and puddings!

Hemp Seeds and Hemp Oil – First, let's be clear that dietary hemp oil will not give you a marijuana "high." Many claim the health benefits of hemp seeds and oil are superior to flax. Hemp seeds are a source of complete protein and hemp oil has a perfect blend of healthy polyunsaturated fats. As with flax, hemp oil and seeds are best when not heated. Enjoy them on salads, add them to smoothies, or top your favorite dish with them. **Bottom Line** - Add variety to your food by including hemp.

Butter (Yes, butter!) – 'Moove' over margarine! Butter is back! With all of the negative publicity about cholesterol and heart disease, butter has had a bad reputation for decades. It is curious that for years we have wondered why the French, whose traditional foods use large amounts of butter, have consistently been leaner and suffered much less heart disease than we Americans. There have been a lot of theories about this, but maybe their butter intake has actually been protective. As it turns out, organic butter from grass fed cows has some amazing health benefits such as: butter contains fat-soluble vitamins A, E and K2. K2 is necessary for heart and bone health. The fat in butter is considered "good fat" and is no longer associated with heart disease or high cholesterol. It has actually been shown to help in weight loss! Wait, there's more – butter also has a special fatty acid called conjugated linoleic acid (CLA), which has been shown to have anti-cancer properties. Also, you can cook with butter without damaging the fat. So sauté away! Best of all, butter is delicious and gives us that comfort food feeling. The key to achieving the most health benefits from butter is using organic butter from grass fed cows. **Bottom Line** - Spread the word; organic butter is good and good for you!

Do Calories Count?

Calories. We have been told for years that the caloric balance equation is the key to weight loss. Most weight loss plans have focused on finding out how many calories are burned and how many are taken in. To lost weight, people should burn more calories than they take in. This has led to a lot of research about "good" calories versus "bad" calories. Recently many top health professionals have delivered the message, "don't focus on calories, instead focus on quality food."

What is the answer, watch calories or focus on quality food? The truth is we have to do both. This what we know about the "bad" calories; those that are not healthful or that have minimal nutritional value:

- They increase fat storage potential;
- They increase risk for inflammatory diseases including heart disease, diabetes, dementia, autoimmune disease and cancer;
- They can keep us feeling hungry and consequently, we eat more.

Good calories on the other hand:

- Calm inflammation;
- Contribute to feeling satisfied and full;
- Allow the body's natural processes to burn fat.

However, the caloric equation is still important. If you take in more calories than you burn, whether they come from good food sources or bad food sources, the balance will tip the scales toward weight gain.

WHEN YOU CAN – GO ORGANIC

Is it worth it to go organic? Absolutely. The most current research has shown that organic foods are more nutritious than conventionally grown foods. If that isn't enough of a reason, here are six more:

- **Toxicity to Earth & Water** - Chemical fertilizers and pesticides harm our environment. These chemicals are known to cause cancer, birth defects and neurological impairment. Bees, which we rely on to pollinate crops and produce food, are becoming endangered, possibly due to the widespread use of pesticides. (Bees travel from field to field and are unable to determine which crops are organic or "conventional".)

- **Cruelty to animals** - "Conventional" practices of raising animals for food involve not only feeding the animal food that is laden with pesticides and herbicides but also hormones, antibiotics and even arsenic. Animals are often maimed, tortured and found wallowing in and ingesting feces.
- **Toxicity to our bodies**- The chemicals that we use in our food supply, our households and in our communities are toxic to our bodies. The human body is an amazing and miraculous collection of systems and functions that work endlessly to keep us well. Over time, with continued bombardment of poisonous compounds, these systems start to fail. Risk of cancer, auto-immune disease and neurological disorders increases with every exposure; every year, every day, every meal, every bite. Yes, every bite counts because it not only presents our bodies with pollutants that must be overcome, but it also contributes to and supports the "mainstream conventional culture."
- **Expense** – Yes, expense. Organics do tend cost a bit more. How can this be a reason to "Go Organic?" Companies and businesses that promote "conventional" food, cleaning supplies, pesticides and fertilizers make their profits betting that people like you and me are more interested in saving money than saving ourselves and the environment. As businesses begin to realize that producing an organic product is what the consumer demands, more and more green companies will emerge and more "conventional" companies will see the wisdom in going green. When this happens, with the power of competition, prices will go down.
- **Tastes Better** – In studies that compared the taste of organic to "conventional" food, including fruit, vegetables, meat and poultry, people consistently preferred the taste of organic food to "conventional" food.
- **Karma** – Whether you believe in Karma or not, the fact is that when you choose organic food and products you are doing good things for you, your family and the planet. The result is a more vibrant and healthful world –both inside the body and out.

Start now. If you are not currently choosing organic or green products, take a look around your home and in your kitchen to see where you can start. Perhaps you will begin by selecting one or two products; those that will make the greatest impact on you and your family. Once you begin to go green, you will find yourself becoming more mindful about the choices you make. Go organic – feel better.

Note: When you see the word "natural" on labels it does not indicate that the product is organic. The word "natural" on a label simply means nothing artificial or synthetic has been added. To be certain you have an organic product, look for the USDA Organic logo.

> *"We do not inherit the earth from our ancestors, we borrow it from our children."*
>
> *~ NATIVE AMERICAN PROVERB*

To Weigh or Not to Weigh? That is the question."

space in your own home. You know what is coming. The dreaded SCALE! As you approach, the memorable theme from "Psycho" is playing through your head, **"screech screech screech screech!"** Oh the terror of getting on a scale. "What will it say?" "What will it tell me about myself?"

> **The Scale:** The Good, the Bad and the Ugly. Not YOU. The SCALE.

> The Good? It's not what the scale says; it is what the scale does. It provides us with an opportunity to see where we are and to track our progress. That's it. No More.

> The Bad? We have to remember that the scale just reports a number. Scale numbers don't portray the composition of our bodies (lean versus fat). The scale doesn't tell us how our clothes are fitting or whether we are less tired at the end of the day.

> The Ugly. Ugly happens when we allow this inanimate object to define our self worth, self image and self esteem. We have to remember that the scale does not judge. It is a tool, like a compass, that we can use to help point us in the right direction.

> So, to Weigh or Not to Weigh? Yes, weigh when you feel the need to check in. But don't allow the scale to hijack your self image or even your good mood. Keep focused on the Good and run like hell from the Ugly!

NOURISHING NOURISHMENT

Tell me what you eat and I will tell you who you are"

~ ANATHELM BRILLAT-SAVARIN

Our relationship with food is integral to our ability to gain and sustain a vital robust body and mind. Our behaviors and feelings about food are so entrenched in who we are and how we interact with friends and family and in social situations that the thought of changing or turning our backs on those behaviors can feel like losing a close friend or loved one. But food, and behaviors around food, that harm us or cause us to feel badly physically or emotionally, will never give us the support we need to reach the level of health and enjoyment that defines a life of wellness.

Supporting yourself, nurturing yourself with wholesome life-giving food is, in fact, giving life to your body, mind and spirit. Each of the billions of your tiny microscopic cells begins to radiate with new energy and light. Even small steps toward making better choices about the food that enters your body will reap benefits. As your whole being begins to receive the gift of healthful nourishment it will thank you with brighter functioning and clearer thinking.

Understanding which foods serve you and which do not is the foundation for choosing wisely. Remember the basics, eat your colors, avoid high glycemic foods, get enough protein for your age and lifestyle, enjoy high quality fats and choose organic unprocessed food when possible. These simple guidelines will help fill in the gray areas where confusion may set in. When in doubt, go back to these guidelines to map out your eating plan. You are in the driver's seat. Enjoy the ride!

Body Wrap

In our Mind section, we talked about wellness in somewhat disembodied terms of thoughts, feelings and behaviors. The concepts in the Three Essentials deal with matters of the Mind, but they are foundational to whole-person health. Once we begin tidying up our *mental* approach to life, we can have a more meaningful conversation about our *physical* selves.

Intellectually we can appreciate the notion of our mental well-being impacting our physical health, but discussing wellness in solely intangible ways is like attempting to go sailing without a boat. Our bodies are the boat. They are the vessels through which our wellness is expressed. Having a clear understanding and direction of how the Three Essentials impact our ability to make good choices, we can enter into the realm of the physical. We can take "OWNership" of our choices based on sound information and begin to make changes in our overall wellness as it is expressed in our bodies.

For many of us, talking about our bodies in a loving and objective way can be difficult. We may be carrying around images of ourselves that are disapproving or disheartening. Or we may have given up and rejected our physical selves altogether. Staying grounded in what we learned in the Mind section, we can accept that we OWN our bodies and have the power to make positive changes in our health and well-being.

OWN is deliberately simple. There is so much information professed in the diet and exercise arena, it can be overwhelming. It may feel like being bogged down in relentless quicksand. No matter how hard you try to get a grip on it and move forward, the uncertainty weighs you down and keeps you stuck in place. OWN simplifies the complicated and often contradictory information and breaks it down into the basics of wellness:

- Breathe. Get more oxygen into your cells. Include mindful movement to enhance the benefits of your oxygen flow.
- Hydrate. Give your body the healthy fluid it needs to carry out all of its essential functions.
- Make better food choices. Give your cells the clean nourishment they need to feed your body and mind.

Seriously. It's that simple. Granted, while it is simple, it may not feel easy. It does require thoughtful decision making and taking action on those decisions. But I will promise you that with every single healthful, positive decision you make, you are taking steps out of the quagmire toward a healthier you, and a lifetime of wellness.

"If we could give every individual the right amount of nourishment and exercise, not too little and not too much, we would have found the safest way to health."

~ *HIPPOCRATES*

Section 3

7

Spirit

annot claim wellness – or even the path to true wellness -without taking steps to cultivate our Spirit. When we nurture our Spirit, we become less anxious, more centered and more conscious of our wellness needs and the choices we must make to attend to those needs. This is why Spirit is foundational to our approach to lifetime wellness.

THE WELLNESS TRINITY – A THREE LEGGED STOOL

Let's imagine wellness as an overarching state of being where all systems are balanced, functioning vibrantly and cooperatively and sustaining harmony in our lives. Utopia! We can easily agree that the Wellness Essentials and OWN contribute to this ideal level of wellness. But without Spirit, our wellness state of being is like a three-legged stool with one leg missing. It is wobbly and out of balance. Wellness consciousness is a trinity of Mind, Body and Spirit. Our indwelling Spirit is entwined in all aspects of our being. We may not always be aware of it, but Spirit is interwoven throughout our everyday lives. The more we kindle this aspect of ourselves, the greater our capacity to achieve balance in the wellness consciousness we seek.

The good news is that everything we have discussed thus far lays the groundwork for cultivating Spirit. The concepts and skills we learned in the Wellness Essentials and

OWN free our Mind and Body to nurture Spirit. These basic needs must be met so that we have the strength and clarity to think about something that seems intangible, like Spirit. When our bodies and minds are stressed, traumatized, thirsty or starving we begin to drift away from our ability to access our Inner Compass. Finding the way back to our Center becomes difficult and sometimes murky. In a very real and tangible sense, caring for our minds and bodies *is elemental* in our ability to attend to Spirit and to enable Spirit to complete our wellness trinity. Each requires the other to be complete. The key to this balance is in our *intention*.

> *"It is more Important to be of pure intention than of perfect action."*
>
> ~ *ILYAS KASSAM*

Intention imparts quality to our purpose or motivation to our actions. To understand what I mean by quality of intention, imagine a person who finds a lost wallet full of cash and dutifully seeks to find the owner and return it, all the while dreaming of his reward; perhaps a portion of the cash that was returned. The owner is thrilled to receive the wallet intact and, indeed offers the finder a small reward. In this scenario, the finder did the "right thing" by returning the wallet. However, the motivation for returning the wallet was to receive a reward. The *quality of the intention* was marred by selfishness. While the finder may be temporarily pleased by the reward, it doesn't provide long-term happiness or a deep sense of contentment.

Now imagine a different scenario in which the finder once again does the "right" thing, finds the owner and returns the wallet intact, motivated solely by the sincere desire to help. In this case the *quality of intention* is wholesome and honorable. The owner is thrilled to receive the wallet and offers the finder a small reward. The finder may or may not accept the award. It doesn't matter. The finder's real satisfaction comes from having connected with what is *true* and *honest* from within himself. The finder was guided by his Inner Compass. He feels complete, satisfied and happy.

When we make an effort to "do the right thing" by caring for ourselves and tending to our minds as with the Three Essentials of Wellness and our bodies as we introduced with OWN, our Spirit responds. Making better choices with food, movement and attitudes resonates with our Inner Compass. Something deep within us knows we are headed in the right direction and begins to light up.

At the same time, the intention with which we make these choices influences our results. When we can mindfully direct the intention of our actions toward feeding our Inner Self, the benefits of our choices increase exponentially. Think of the metaphor of the pebble in the pond. When we toss a small pebble into the quiet waters of the pond, no doubt there is a ripple effect, with ringlets of water moving outward from the place the pebble plopped in. But if we were to take a large stone and throw it forcefully (yet lovingly) into the pond, we would create quite a splash, perhaps creating wavelets rather than ringlets. These examples illustrate different levels, or quality, of intention. The intention behind the act of throwing the stone determines the magnitude of the result. Using this metaphor, our Inner Self is the quiet pond and our intention to nurture ourselves is the gusto with which we make better choices.

Can you recall a beloved teacher you had in school; one you vividly remember for making the subject matter come alive for you? What did that feel like for you? Did it invigorate your enthusiasm for the subject? Does the memory still make you smile and appreciate that teacher? The wonderful teacher that stands out in my memory is Mrs. Shelley who taught English literature. I will always remember how this spindly, gray-haired, polio survivor would become vividly animated describing a Victorian novel in a way that could wake up even the most dormant teenager. Her blue eyes danced us across England's heath with such excitement; it delights me even today to remember her.

On the other hand, did you ever have a teacher who simply opened the book and read in a monotone; or put the lesson on the chalkboard and left it to you to figure out? If so, I suspect you don't have wonderful memories of that teacher, or the subject for that matter.

In these examples both teachers share the intention of conveying the required material to the student. But one had a much higher quality of intention. That greater intention made waves. It produced a greater, more positive, long-lasting and profound impact on the intended result. The same is true when the quality of our intention to nurture ourselves with healthy Mind and Body practices is genuine and sincere.

111

I once worked with a lovely young woman whom I always admired for her commitment to a healthy lifestyle. I remember once seeing her unpack her lunch. As she described all the nutritious food in her lunch she became more and more illumined, until she at last beamed, "I love this! It is so good for me!" She was consciously and intentionally loving her Self; not just her body and her mind, but also her Inner Self. She glowed.

We can see that using the power of quality intention, we can significantly enhance our feelings of wellness and well-being. The intention to evoke our Inner Self is something we can bring to everything that we do. Whether it is making good decisions about nourishing our bodies, moving mindfully, caring for our families, attending to work, completing daily tasks or simply unpacking our lunch, this attention to our Spirit balances our wellness consciousness by magnifying the good in whatever we do.

HOW DO WE "EVOKE" OUR INNER SELF?

Approach life situations (e.g. family, work, rest, play, problems) with love. Take the tools you have already practiced in mindfulness and compassion and add a touch of love. We are not talking about romantic love. We are talking about the kind of love you have for a child, a pet, art, nature or music; the kind of love that stirs your soul or makes your Inner Self smile. This kind of love expresses itself in kindness, patience, consideration and benevolence. It allows your Spirit to connect with an everyday situation and elevate it to a meaningful experience.

Foster sincerity in your interactions with others. Sincerity requires that we recognize and acknowledge the honesty of our Inner Self and express that outwardly and with kindness. Too often we try "to be" something we are not. Maybe we want to appear smarter, stronger, more attractive or "cool". When we do this we are actually withholding our Inner Self from the situation. When we allow the genuineness of our true nature to shine through, our interactions are less stressful and result in a more positive outcome.

Express Gratitude. Being thankful for the myriad experiences in our lives begins with being mindfully aware; noticing the wonders that occur in our lives everyday and over time. Dr. Robert Emmons, a leading researcher on gratitude, explains that gratitude is a way of thinking about receiving a benefit and acknowledging someone or something outside of ourselves for that benefit. Making a gratitude list will change your life. Dr. Emmons explains that developing gratitude helps us to take things *"as granted"* rather than *"for granted"*. This simple practice helps us feel energetic, alive, connected to the world around us and has even been shown to improve academic performance. When we begin to practice gratitude we may find that expressing gratitude is like peeling an onion; we have superficial layers, such as "grateful for my home", but as we peel away the layers we may find we are thankful for our life experiences that brought us to this home, for the view outside of the kitchen window, for the warmth of the sun as we sit in our favorite chair and for a place to feel safe and loved at the end of the day. As we peel the layers further and further we discover our gratitude both magnifies and amplifies. It reverberates within us. If you have never practiced writing a gratitude list, perhaps now would be a good time to try. If you have done this before – GREAT! Let's do it again – and as often as possible.

PRACTICE

Take a moment now. In the space below, write down at least five things for which you are grateful. You might start each entry with "I am grateful for..." As you write each one down, pause to think about why you are grateful. Focus on peeling away the layers, going deeper with each entry. What can you name that you are grateful for this very day? What qualities does each entry possess that gives you the feeling of gratitude? As you do this exercise, notice your sense of happy calm growing from within.

1.
2.
3.
4.
5.

Each time you connected to the essence of your gratitude, how did you feel?Joyful? Serene? Delighted? These feelings represent the connection to your Spirit. For best results, make a gratitude list at least once per week. Of course, finding moments in everyday to pause for gratitude will really boost your benefits.

Gratitude can transform common days into thanksgivings, turn routine jobs into joy, and change ordinary opportunities into blessings.

~ WILLIAM ARTHUR WARD

Itadakimasu!

The Japanese have a lovely tradition of saying the word "Itadakimasu" (Eee-tah-dah-kee-mahs) before a meal. Some mistakenly loosely translate the word to something similar to "Bon Appetit", or "Let's Eat." But Itadakimasu is actually a profound term that expresses gratitude. Itadakimasu reflects the principle of respecting all living things. Saying Itadakimasu conveys grati-tude to the plants and animals that gave their lives for the meal, as well as all concerned in providing the meal, from the hunter, fisher or farmer to the preparer. Itadakimasu is great way to connect with your Spirit and acknowledge the Spirit of all who are contributing to your nourishment. It is properly said with the hands clasped and a slight bow, but I like to say it with enthusiasm, as thought it were a toast, "Itadakimasu!"

WELLNESS FROM THE IN-SIDE OUT - CONNECTING WITH YOUR INNER SELF

"The quieter you become the more you can hear"

~ RAM DAS

As we deepen our discussion on Spirit and Wellness, it might help to think about our conversations in the Mind and Body portions of the book as wellness from the outside effecting change on the inside. In those discussions we considered our feelings about ourselves and others, we encouraged our breath and nurtured our bodies with healthful food and hydration. We know that doing these things will restore health to all the systems in our bodies and that this health will be reflected in how we experience life.

Now that we have come to our discussion on Spirit, we are looking at wellness from the inside influencing change on the outside, or wellness from the in-side out. We tiptoed into this idea in our earlier conversation about mindful awareness. There we discussed ways in which we can practice being attentively present and we listed many of the physiological and psychological benefits of practicing mindfulness. Here we begin to wade in a little deeper. When we begin to practice mindful awareness in our daily lives something amazing happens; we open the channel that connects our outer awareness to our Inner Self.

As we become more and more aware of this channel and seek to navigate this connection with intention, we have access to our Source or Inner Compass. This *effort to connect* is generally termed "meditation." Along with all the benefits of mindfulness, "meditation" can enhance our sense of calm, inner peace and happiness. It boosts creativity and sharpens focus. And because we are accessing our Inner Compass, our intuition sharpens. We have a sense of direction.

Here again it is important to remember our definition of Wellness, *"...the natural mix of elements that make us unique."* How each of us chooses to connect with our Source or Inner Self is as unique as we are ourselves. Truly, if you do not have a regular practice of connecting, the hardest part is getting started.

When I was in the early stages of my personal inner journey, my daughter – the eldest of two children – was in high school. I had been reading about meditation and trying to practice occasionally when I had quiet moments alone on nature walks or hikes of some sort. When I finally decided I would commit to a daily meditation practice, I waited until my daughter was headed off to school in the morning. I thought practicing by the fireplace in our living room would be nice, so I took a book of beginning meditations, went into the living room and quietly settled in to attempt a few minutes of "real meditation." About that time my daughter came bursting back into the house. She had forgotten something. She saw me seated there and said in her fully teen-aged high school voice, *"What* are you doing?" Frustrated and exasperated, I replied, "I am *trying* to *meditate*." She flipped around to go back out the door, tossing her head and said, "You are SO weird!" That was the end of meditating in the living room. So, I carved out a small space in my bedroom where I could go at any time, but most typically in the morning before my daughter woke up!

Most of us resist the idea of "meditation". "I am too busy", we complain. Sitting still and not "being productive" feels like a complete waste of our precious time. What are we supposed to do while we sit there? Is there a right way? "Listen to what I have to say!", the mind continually nags. That voice in our head keeps yammering away no matter how hard we try to shush it. Our minds churn and our resistance intensifies.

Some people find the term "meditation" off-putting. If the idea of "meditation" feels like it is not your cup of tea, think of it in other terms, such as; quiet time, time out, or "me-time". Whatever you choose to call it and however you choose to do it, taking a few moments (or more if you can) to quiet your mind and your breath will allow you to go inward and commune with your Source.

I believe that a meditation practice is simply about taking a few minutes on a regular basis to connect to your Inner Source. Because we are all different, we have to find our own path inward. People who struggle with sitting still may need to do a walking meditation, or a moving meditation through dance. Others may prefer to connect to their Spirit in nature or through music. Once you have found your personal ability to connect, you might begin to find that you can access your Inner Self at various times throughout the day; sort of like checking your compass to make sure your are headed in the right direction.

"In the midst of movement and chaos, keep stillness inside of you."

~ DEEPAK CHOPRA

"Turn up the corners" Can smiling be meditative?
The next time you are in a busy place with lots of people, take a moment to observe, without judgment, their facial expressions. You will likely notice that many people wear a permanent frown, or a "turning down" of the corners of their lips. It appears to me that over time, faces begin to get stuck that way. If you are fortunate to see someone who is happily enjoying the moment, notice how free and luminous he or she seems. Maybe just looking at them makes you feel happier and more contented too. Smiling is good for you and good for the people around you. Try it now. It doesn't have to be a big toothy smile. Simply turn up the corners of your lips.

Feeling better yet?

Taoists perform a smiling "meditation." In his book *Being Peace*, Tich Nhat Hahn reminds us that smiling makes us the master of ourselves. Consider the beginning phrase of a smile meditation:

"Breathing in, I calm body and mind
Breathing out, I smile."

LETTING THE LARGER EMERGE

Let's take another look at our wellness quote:

"Wellness - It's the best in each of us, a natural mix of elements that makes us unique. Wellness is a conscious commitment to growth and improvement in all areas. <u>Only then does the larger picture emerge</u>."

~ ANONYMOUS

This is where the "larger picture" emerges. All of the elements in the Mind and Body sections that we have talked about thus far are like pixels or brush stokes in the portrait of our lives. Each of these elements is like a point in a dot-to-dot or paint-by-numbers kit. They give us a general, recognizable outline or image of the vision we have for ourselves. Spirit synergistically blends the individual parts together, revealing the whole; rendering the "larger picture" of our vision. The result is a masterpiece created by our unique desire and ability to enrich our lives.

More "Connection" Activities

This list of simple suggestions will help you develop an awareness of connecting with your Inner Self.

1. Create A Connection Journal. For many of us it is helpful to write down our feelings, observations and questions in a place they can be saved and returned to at a later date. Your Connection Journal is not necessarily a diary but a way to access and begin to connect, or converse, with your Inner Self. One famous example is the "Conversations With God" series of books by Neal Donald Walsch in which Mr. Walsch documents his questions and concerns about life and discovers answers through his connection to his Source. We may not have the same experience as Mr. Walsch, but journaling can open channels of communication that allow inner wisdom to emerge outwardly in our daily lives. Over time you may go back to entries in your Connection Journal and find that you have experienced profound areas of personal growth, or that questions that may have troubled you in the past have either eased or have been answered.

2. Select a Spirit Mantra to help connect before entering into situations you anticipate will be stressful, such as a meeting with an employer/employee,

travel or doctor's visit. Spirit Mantra is a technique that uses a repeated phrase to connect to our Inner Source and focuses on a positive outcome. It can be of any length and you may find several that you like to use, depending on the situation. I found one I like that was attached to a Reiki candle: "May light and love surround and protect me in all my endeavors." Here is another one adapted from Ernest Holmes, "Within myself I find the guidance and strength I need." Or maybe something like this from Og Mandino, "I greet this day with love in my heart." You can use these or create or one of your own. Be on the lookout. As you begin to connect more frequently, Spirit Mantras will appear in all kinds of places. Write down those that you find inspiring and keep them somewhere you can refer back to.

3. Engage in body-gratification reflection. Sit or lay quietly and allow your breath to settle down. In your mind's eye, take a moment and focus on a specific part of your body, consider all that this part does for you throughout your day, everyday, and send gratitude to that part. You can begin with your feet, moving up through legs and arms. Include your heart and lungs as well as other organs such as your digestive organs and even your skin. Thank your brain, tongue and vocal chords for thought, taste and speech. Thank your eyes and ears for the ability to see the goodness in life and hear the sounds of nature and joy.

4. Each day make a conscious effort to recognize everyday beauty. Noticing the beauty in ordinary occurrences helps us to see extraordinary events that we may otherwise pass by. This recognition and appreciation connects us directly to our Source. Look around. You may observe children laughing and playing, a bird's nest, plants emerging from the winter into new growth, colorful umbrellas on a rainy day, snow blanketed mountains and trees, the warmth of the sun, a cool breeze on your skin or the multitude of colors that embellish a landscape. You can find hundreds of occasions to recognize beauty each day. The idea is to simply STOP, NOTICE, RECOGNIZE and APPRECIATE.

5. Make a joyful noise. Singing, humming and chanting are effective ways to connect your inner and outer wellness. Each of these help produce a sense of happiness and well-being – and you don't even need to be on key! The sounds and vibrations of singing, chanting and particularly humming induce

relaxation, reduce blood pressure and respiration rate, clear the mind and improve depression. What a great reason to sing in the shower, hum a favorite tune (or even hum as you exhale), learn a beloved Buddhist chant, such as Om, or belt out a tune with the radio in your car. The key is to bring it forth from the joy in your heart!

THE SPIRIT OF WELLNESS

When we talk about "Sprit" in the context of our journey toward lifetime wellness, we are talking about our connection to our own divine nature and the recognition of that divinity in others and in our surroundings. Developing a sense of spiritual connection can help us cope with stressful situations, enhance our ability to relax, improve our ability to heal and enhance our personal sense of calm. These things are integral to our ability to experience whole-person wellness.

In essence, we can begin to see that the path to wellness can also be considered a spiritual path. As we tend to Mind, Body and Sprit, we begin to see that these are not separate entities, but one interconnected wonderful being – YOU. Caring for any aspect of Mind, Body or Spirit, we can't help but influence our wellness as a whole being. When you nurture your Inner Self by approaching life with love, sincerity and gratitude, you actually *become* a "Well Being."

"Spiritual practice is returning again and again to softness."

~ STEPHANIE DOWRICK

Section 4

8

Stepping Stones

"No one saves us but ourselves. No one can and no one may. We ourselves must walk the path."

~ BUDDHA

We have come to the end of this conversation, but our journey together is not over. The knowledge you have gained and the practices you have begun are stepping-stones on your journey toward Lifetime Wellness. You have come a long way thus far. Let's take a look.

You have reconnected with your self esteem and self efficacy. Perhaps your self respect has seen a boost since you have been applying some of the information you have received in this book. You have begun to heal your mind and body though the use of positive words, images and mindfulness. You have learned the importance of breath and that your body needs to move and be free. You have started to include more water and health giving foods in your daily routine and perhaps have also reduced or eliminated many of the foods that are not supportive in your quest for wellness. Finally, you have explored a relationship with your Source to help discover your inner compass and provide guidance along your journey.

At last it's time to create a personal road map that will direct your next steps on your journey. But before you embark, there are Three Keys to Success that will help you overcome obstacles you will encounter along the way. Keep them with you to help you remain steadfast in your quest toward Lifetime Wellness.

THE THREE KEYS TO SUCCESS
Key #1 Courage

> *"God grant us the serenity to accept the things we cannot change, courage to change the things we can, and wisdom to know the difference."*
>
> *~ REINHOLD NIEBUHR*

One would hardly imagine that making the decision to be better, feel better - more whole - would require courage. But the fact is, change is hard. We all face change in every aspect of our lives. We experience change at work, in our families, our friends and the world around us. The ironic thing about change is that it is constant.

How we cope with change affects our overall health and well-being. Change can cause worry, anxiety and stress. We can choose to allow change to overwhelm our emotions and take our well-being hostage or we can make the choice to see change as simply a part of life and recognize that while we may not have the ability to prevent change, we absolutely have the power to control our response to it.

Now here you are. You have chosen to read this book and do some, if not all, of the practices. This means that you are, at the very least, contemplating change. You are making the decision to look at your current state of health and wellness and to begin a journey that can guide you to improved health, enhanced well-being and increased self-efficacy.

When we begin to make lifestyle changes, it is not only uncomfortable for us personally; it is uncomfortable for those around us - family, friends, even co-workers. Why? Because over the course of our lives, we have developed an identity. This identity is how people know us. We could say they "identify" us in a certain way or actually may even "identify with" us. As we begin to change, those people with whom we have relationships may feel uncomfortable about the changes taking place. Some people may be confused about the decisions we make. They may not understand why we have made these choices. They may ridicule, make fun, or even reject us for the choices we have made to change our lives. To stay the course, to hold onto our convictions, to continue our quest, we must have courage. As we begin to incorporate mindfulness into our day and recognize the hundreds of choices that can impact our well-being, we will need courage to make the choice that is best for us, even if others do not understand. In some cases, we may even need the courage to say good-bye.

"Courage does not always roar. Sometimes courage is the quiet voice at the end of the day saying, 'I will try again tomorrow."

~ MARY ANNE RADMACHER

Key #2 Resilience

The next Key goes hand-in-hand with courage. *Resilience*. Resilience is that quality that enables us to emerge from difficult situations with the ability to persevere. With resilience we learn from our mistakes and, along with courage, resolve to make a better choice next time. When we have a clear sense of purpose and a vision for our future, resilience is the part of our character that enables us to bounce back from setbacks and facilitates our commitment to growth. Remember our definition of Wellness?

"Wellness is a conscious commitment to growth and improvement in all areas. "

Do not judge me by my successes, judge me by how many times I fell down and got back up again."

~ NELSON MANDELA

Key #3 Determination

The third Key is *Determination*. Determination is about having the drive to succeed. It is strongly related to desire. In our previous discussions you have envisioned a future for yourself, your health and your well-being. You are learning to be mindful of that vision; beginning to feel it, taste it and express it in your daily life. You *desire* it. The path to your success will be beset with obstacles. You may have the courage to face them, the resilience to overcome them, but to achieve success you must also have the determination to keep moving, even if it is baby steps, toward the vision of your future.

You desire an outcome, a lifestyle, a state of physical and mental wellness. Allow your desire to strengthen your determination. Begin to recognize your resilience and applaud it. Look back at each obstacle you have overcome and honor it for providing you with opportunity for growth and the realization of the *New You* that you desire.

> *"Never give in. Never give in. Never, never, never, never—in nothing, great or small, large or petty—never give in, except to convictions of honour and good sense."*
>
> *~ WINSTON S. CHURCHILL*

LET'S TAKE A MOMENT NOW TO RECONSIDER YOUR WELLNESS RULER

Recall that the left side of the ruler might contain words such as:

Lethargic

Weary

Stressed

Overwhelmed

Powerless

The right side of the ruler might include words such as:

Buoyant

Zestful

Vitality

Enthusiastic

Excited

Possible descriptors for points between 1 and 10 include:

From 2-4:

Dull

Indifferent

Unmotivated

Weak

Lack luster

From 4-6

Accepting

Considering

Reasonable

Satisfactory

From 7-9

Energetic

Optimistic

Positive

Confident

Thinking about all that you have learned and practiced thus far, make a point at which you find yourself now and add words that describe the point you selected.

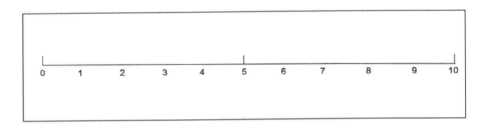

Where did you place yourself on the Wellness Ruler the first time? The second time?

Do you recall the vision you created for yourself in the first Wellness Essential and how you envisioned your life when you selected your first two points on the Wellness Ruler? What has changed for you? How has the knowledge you have gained or the modifications you have made, influenced how you feel?

Knowing that you have the foundation to make healthful choices and the power to set your life journey in the direction of wellness, take a moment now to refine the vision of yourself. Include vivid descriptions including feelings, sensations, relation-ships, and body image.

My Vision for Myself and My life:

"Be patient with yourself. Self-growth is tender; it's holy ground. There's no greater investment."

~ STEPHEN COVEY

NEXT STEPS

Now it is time to map out your plan for the next steps on your journey. Sit quietly for a few moments (or as long as it takes) and consider what actions you can take that will move you forward toward Lifetime Wellness. Below, you will find space to list actions that you can take daily, weekly, or monthly as well as a space to record what you intend to achieve by taking these actions. You will also find a list of suggestions for each area. These are only suggestions; perhaps they will spur you to come up with some of your own.

DAILY

Suggestions
Daily:
Drink at least 60 ounces of water.

Take at least 5 – 10 minutes to begin a "Connection Practice."

Set a timer and plan to get up from the chair or workspace and incorporate movement at least 5 times per day.

Plan healthy meal and snack choices.

Choose organic food when possible.

MY PLAN:

WEEKLY

Suggestions
Weekly:

Exercise at least 3-5 times per week for a total of 90-150 minutes.

Locate and attend a local grower's market.

Spend quality activity time with your children and/or spouse.

Spend time in a beautiful natural setting, such as a park or nature center.

Write a gratitude list.

MY PLAN:

MONTHLY

Suggestions
Monthly:
Read a book on a wellness topic.

Watch a documentary on food and health.

Find and practice a wellness CD or DVD on exercise or meditation. (Check out the resource page for ideas.)

Review how your plan is going and revise as necessary for success!

Check in with your Wellness Ruler to track your progress.

MY PLAN:

OTHER IDEAS AND SUGGESTIONS:

Meet with a nationally certified fitness professional to help develop a personalized exercise program. You may need to meet only occasionally to get guidelines for safe exercise or you may choose to meet frequently so that the trainer can monitor and modify your routine as necessary.

Meet with a certified nutritionist, certified health coach or licensed dietitian to review and help revise your eating plan. Once again, this does not have to be on-going, but it can provide an opportunity to find areas in your eating plan that are not working for you and to offer better options.

Make a contract with yourself to accomplish the items in your plan. Your contract could look something like this:

By committing to and successfully completing the items in this plan, I will achieve:
(write your specific intentions here)

I understand it will take time to fully accomplish these objectives and I will establish reasonable expectations. I will frequently review my progress and will adjust my course as necessary with compassion, courage, resilience and determination.

Your name_____

Date _____

> *"Do not sit still; start moving now. In the beginning, you may not go in the direction you want, but as long as you are moving, you are creating alternatives and possibilities."*
>
> *~ RODOLFO COSTA*

THE IMPORTANCE OF YOUR VISION

Throughout the ages, sages have told us that the reality we desire actually exists within us. We don't have to evolve into it. Like Dorothy, we have to make the twisting, turning journey toward Oz until at last we realize that we have what we were seeking all along. We just need to recognize it.

Therefore, create your Vision with clarity and confidence. Be clear in your quest. Bring forth the greater good that is within you. Stick to your vision and don't be dissuaded or discouraged.

"Trust yourself. You know more than you think you do."

~ BENJAMIN SPOCK

As you continue on your path, like Dorothy, you will be confronted with difficult choices and intimidating circumstances. When these things happen, remember your vision with utmost precision, access your inner compass and use the tools you have been given in this book to help you take the steps that will keep you headed in the right direction.

Remember that change is not easy and can be scary, especially when we are working to change ideas and behaviors that have been ingrained in us since birth. Sometimes it can feel as though we are turning our back on our upbringing, the comfort we find in our already established lifestyles and perhaps even people we love. But the truth is, we are turning our hearts toward health, well-being and happiness, which is our true nature.

"What the caterpillar calls the end of the world, the master calls a butterfly. "

~ RICHARD BACH

FINAL THOUGHTS

As we continue to choose a lifestyle of wellness thoughts and actions, we begin to impact not only our own lives, but also the lives of those around us: our spouses, children, friends, neighbors and our communities. We effectively become "the pebble in the pond." Our wellness expands outward. Isn't it beautiful that by healing ourselves we can also heal the people and the planet we love? And so it is my friend, together, step-by-step and hand-in-hand, we begin to heal our world.

"Act as if what you do makes a difference. It does."

~ WILLIAM JAMES

RESOURCES FOR WELLNESS
Healthy Food
Seek:

> Local Harvest localharvest.org
> Eat Wild eatwild.com
> USDA.gov/amsv1.0farmersmarkets (check on this)
> Eat Well Guide Eatwellguide.org
> Food Routes foodroutes.org
> ChooseMyPlate.gov

Read:

> "Wheat Belly", William Davis M.D.
> "Grain Brain", David Pulmutter M.D.
> "Gut Bliss", Robynne Chutkin M.D.
> "The Skinny on Fats", David Brownstein M.D.
> "Eat Fat Get Thin", Mark Hyman M.D.

Watch:

> "Fed Up"

Mindfulness
Read:

> "The Four Agreements", Don Miguel Ruiz
> "Mindfulness to Go", David Harp M.A.
> "Loving Yourself to Great Health", Louise Hay, Ahlea Khadro, Heather Dane
> "Words Can Change Your Brain", Andrew Newberg M.D., Mark Robert Waldman
> "Mindsight", Daniel Siegel M.D.

"Be Here Now", Ram Das
"The Power of Now", Eckhart Tolle
"Practicing the Presence", Joel S. Goldsmith
https://www.psychologytoday.com/blog/some-assembly-required/201404/what-constitutes-spiritual-awakening

Listen:

"Headspace", Meditation made simple, https://www.headspace.com

Breath

Read:

"How God Changes Your Brain", Andrew Newberg M.D. and Mark Robert Waldman
"Buddha's Brain", Rick Hanson PhD, Richard Mendius M.D.
"Breathing: The Master Key to Self Healing", Andrew Weil M.D.

Listen:

"Breathing: A Beginner's Guide to Increased Health and Vitality", Ken Cohen

Movement

Watch, Read & Do
"foundations of pilates" DVD, Mary Jayne Rogers Ph.D. http://www.doctor-maryjayne.com/categories-listing/instructional-dvd
"Mindful Movements: Ten Exercises for Well-Being", Thich Nhat Hanh
"Get Up! Why Your Chair Is Killing You and What You Can Do About It", James A. Levine
"8 Steps to a Pain Free Back", Esther Gokhale L.Ac.
"Deskbound: Sitting is the New Smoking", Kelly Starrett Ph.D.

Seek More

Consumer Wellness Center http://www.consumerwellness.org
GreenMedInfo Education Equals Empowerment http://www.greenmedinfo.
com
Robert Wood Johnson Foundation http://www.rwjf.org
Healthy Eating Research http://healthyeatingresearch.org
Physician's Committee for Responsible Medicine http://pcrm.org
Environmental Working Group http://www.ewg.org
Institute for Responsible Technology http://responsibletechnology.org
Earth Open Source http://earthopensource.org
Center for Science in the Public Interest http://cspinet.org

Index of Authors' Quotes

I hope the quotes I have selected along the way have helped to motivate, inspire or make you smile. Please see the index below for more information about the authors*.

Goethe ~ Johann Wolfgang von Goethe (1749-1832) Writer, poet, scientist, statesman

Lao Tzu ~ Ancient Chinese philosopher andw. Author of Tao Te Ching and father of Toaism

Plato ~ Classical Greece Philosopher

James Gordon ~ Author, poet, composer, artist

George Bernard Shaw ~ (1856-1950) Irish playwright and critic. Awarded the Nobel Prize in Literature in 1925.

Buddha ~ Guatama Buddha. Ascetic and sage upon whose teachings Buddhism was founded.

Golda Meir ~ (1898-1978) Israeli stateswoman, politician and the fourth Prime Minister of Isreal.

Ralph Waldo Emerson ~ (1803-1882) American essayist, lecturer and poet.

Carl Jung ~ Carl Gustave Jung (1875-1961) Swiss psychiatrist and psychotherapist who founded analytical psychology.

Henepola Gunaratana ~ Bhante Henepola Gunaratana is a Sri Lankan Theravada Buddhist monk.

Eleanor Roosevelt ~ Anna Eleanor Roosevelt (1884-1962). American politician, diplomat and activist. Longest serving First Lady of the United States.

Thich Nhat Hanh ~ Vietnamese Buddist monk, teacher, author, poet and peace activist.

Jon Kabat-Zinn ~ Professor of Medicine Emeritus, founder of the Stress Reduction Clinic and Center for Mindfulness in Medicine, Health Care, and Society at the University of Massachusetts Medical School.

Kate Wicker ~ "wife, mom, author, & speaker"

Brene Brown ~ American scholar, author, public speaker and research professor at the University of Houston Graduate College of Social Work.

Henry David Thoreau ~ (1817-1862) American author, poet, philosopher, abolitionist, naturalist, surveyor and historian.

Joseph Hubertus Pilates ~ (1883- 1967) German born physical trainer, author and father of the Pilates method of exercise.

Chandogya Upanishad ~ A Sanskrit text embedded in the Sama Veda of Hinduism. One of the oldest of the 108 Upanishads.

Mark Twain ~ Samuel Langhorne Clemens (1835-1910) American author and humorist.

Ernest Holmes ~ Ernest Shrtleff Homes (1887-1960) American New Thought writer, teacher and leader. Founded the spiritual New Thought movement and the philosophy of "The Science of Mind".

Dave Barry ~ David McAlisterBarry is an American Pulitzer Prize winning author and columnist.

Haruki Murakami ~ Contemporary Japanese author.

Hippocrates ~ (460 BC- 370 BC) Greek physician of the Age of Pericles; referred to as the "Father of Wester Medicine".

From Overwhelmed to Inspired

Gregory Maguire ~ American Novelist.

Leonardo da Vinci ~ Leonardo di ser Piero da Vinci (1452-1519) Italian genius in the areas of invention, paining, sculpting, architecture, science music, mathematics, literature, anatomy geology, astronomy. cartography, engineering, history and botany.

Albert Szent-Gyorgyi ~ (1893-1986) Hungarian American Nobel Prize winning physiologist credited for the discovery of Vitamin C.

Loren Eiseley ~ (1970- 1977) American anthropologist, educator, philosopher, and natural science writer.

Leena Arif

Buddy Hackett ~ (1924-2003) American comedian and actor.

Lucille Ball ~ Lucille Desire Ball (1911-1989) American actress, comedian, model, film executive and producer.

Marianne Williamson ~ American spiritual teacher, author and lecturer.

Beth McCollister

Seneca ~ Lucious Seneca Annaeus (4 BC – 65 AD) Roman philosopher, statesman, dramatist and humorist.

Anais Nin ~ (1903-1977) French essayist and memoirist.

Og Mandino ~ Augustine Mandino (1923-1996) American author.

Anthelm Brillat-Savarin ~ Jean Anthelm Brillat-Savarin (1755-1826) French lawyer and politician famous for his love of food. Founded the gastromic essay.

Ilyas Kassam ~ Author, philosopher, chef.

William Arthur Ward ~ (1921-1994) American author, poet and columnist.

Ram Das ~ American spiritual teacher and author.

Deepak Chopra ~ Indian American physician, author, public speaker and founder of The Chopra Foundation.

Stephanie Dowrick ~ Reverend Dr. Stephanie Dowrick. New Zealand Australian author.

Reinhold Niebuhr ~ (1892-1971) American theologian.

Mary Anne Radmacher ~ Author, artist and professional speaker.

Nelson Mandela ~ Nelson Rolihlahla Mandela (1918-2013) South African anti-apartheid revolutionary, politician and philanthropist who served as President of South Africa from 1994-1999.

Winston S. Churchill ~ Sir Winston Leonard Spencer-Churchill (18714-1965) British who statesman who served as Prime Minister of the United Kingdom from 1940-1945 and again from 1951-1955.

Stephen Covey ~ (1932-2012) American educator, author, businessman and keynote speaker.

Rodolfo Costa ~ Peruvian American author.

Benjamin Spock ~ Benjamin McLane Spock (1903-1998) American pediatrician, author and activist.

Richard Bach ~ American author best known for his metaphorical book "Jonathan Livingston Seagull.

William James ~ (1842-1910) American philosopher, psychologist and physician, has been described as the Father of American Psychology.

*Thank you to Wikipedia for author information.

References

Cherry, Kendra (December 17, 2015). What is Self-Efficacy? Retrieved from http://psychology.about.com/od/theoriesofpersonality/a/self_efficacy.htm

Stanford School of Medicine, The Center for Compassion and Altruism REseach and Education Retrieved from http://ccare.stanford.edu/research/peer-reviewed-ccare-articles/

University of California Berkeley, The Greater Good Science Center, Retrieved from http://greatergood.berkeley.edu/topic/compassion/definition

How Stress Affects the Body, (March 31, 2014) Retrieved from http://www.heartmath.com/infographics/how-stress-affects-the-body/

Babauta, Leo (August 12, 2011) The Amazing Power of Being Present. Retrieved from http://zenhabits.net/mindful/

Davis, Daphne M. and Hayes, Jeffery A. (July/August 2012, Vol. 43, No. 7) Retrieved from http://www.apa.org/monitor/2012/07-08/ce-corner.aspx

Zarcone, Kelly. Mindfulness Training Has Positive Health Benefits. Retrieved from http://nau.edu/Research/Feature-Stories/Mindfulness-Training-Has-Positive-Health-Benefits/

What are the Health Benefits of Mindfulness? Retrieved from https://www.brown.edu/campus-life/health/services/promotion/general-health-emotional-health/mindfulness

Scott, Elizabeth. (December 4, 2014) Mindfulness: The Health and Stress Relief Benefits. Retrieved from http://stress.about.com/od/tensiontamers/a/mindfulness.htm

Bradberry, Travis. (October 8, 2014) Multitasking Damages Your Brain And Career, New Studies Suggest. Retrieved from http://www.forbes.com/sites/travisbradberry/2014/10/08/multitasking-damages-your-brain-and-career-new-studies-suggest/

Small, Gary. Is Multitasking Bad for the Brain? Retrieved from http://bigthink.com/videos/is-multitasking-bad-for-the-brain

Schuder, Kirsten. Psychological Responses to Stress. Retrieved from http://stress.lovetoknow.com/Physiological_Responses_to_Stress

Stress effects on the body. Retrieved from http://www.apa.org/helpcenter/stress-body.aspx

Mohd, Razali Salleh. (Malaysian Journal of Medical Sciences, October, 2008, 15(4). Retrieved from http://www.ncbi.nlm.nih.gov/pmc/articles/PMC3341916/

Stress (January 30, 2013) Retrieved from http://umm.edu/health/medical/reports/articles/stress

Managing Stress. Retrieved from http://www.cmhc.utexas.edu/stress.html

Kunst, Jennifer. (September 2011) Three Fingers Pointing Back to You: Why we see the bad in other rather than ourselves. Retrieved from https://www.psychology-today.com/blog/headshrinkers-guide-the-galaxy/201109/three-fingers-pointing-back-you

Relaxation techniques: Breath control helps quell errant stress response. Retrieved from http://www.health.harvard.edu/mind-and-mood/relaxation-techniques-breath-control-helps-quell-errant-stress-response

Lewis, Dennis. Articles and Essays. Retrieved from http://www.dennislewis.org/articles-other-writings/articles-essays/

Newberg, Andrew and Waldman, Mark Robert. "How God Changes Your Brain". (2009).

United States Geological Survey. The USGS Water Science School. Retrieved from http://water.usgs.gov/edu/propertyyou.html

http://www.ncbi.nlm.nih.gov/pmc/articles/PMC3428767/

Gray, Michael. (Cold Spring Harbor Perspectives in Biology, September 2012, 4(9)) Retrieved from http://www.ncbi.nlm.nih.gov/pmc/articles/PMC3428767/

Kravitz, Len. Water. The Science of Nature's Most Important Nutrient. Retrieved from http://www.drlenkravitz.com/Articles/waterDLK.html

Panel on Dietary Reference Intakes for Electrolytes and Water; Standing Committee on the Scientific Evaluation of Dietary Reference Intakes; Food and Nutrition Board; Institute of Medicine. Retrieved from http://www8.nationalacademies.org/onpinews/newsitem.aspx?RecordID=10925

Wikipedia. Gastrocolic Reflex. Retrieved from https://en.wikipedia.org/wiki/Gastrocolic_reflex

Kilgour, Govan. The health benefits of drinking water are innumerable. Retrieved from http://www.secrets-of-longevity-in-humans.com/benefits-of-drinking-water.html

Primack, Jeff. "Conquering Any Disease". 2012.

Kim, Young, Schutzler, Scott, Schrader, Amy, Spencer, Horace et al., Quantitiy of dietary protein intake, but not pattern of intake, affects net protein balance primarily through differences in protein synthesis in older adults. American Journal of Physiology - Endocrinology and Metabolism (December 2014) Vol. 308 no. 1 Retrieved from http://ajpendo.physiology.org/content/308/1/E21

Benjamin Franklin the Autobiography and Other Writings. Retrieved from http://www.flamebright.com/PTPages/Benjamin.asp

Muth, Natalie Digate. Application of Nutrition. ACE Health Coach Manual (2013).

48963950R00094

Made in the USA
San Bernardino, CA
09 May 2017